**Eleventh International
Congress of Anatomy, Part A**

GLIAL AND NEURONAL
CELL BIOLOGY

PROGRESS IN CLINICAL AND BIOLOGICAL RESEARCH

Series Editors   Vincent P. Eijsvoogel   Seymour S. Kety
Nathan Back   Robert Grover   Sidney Udenfriend
George J. Brewer   Kurt Hirschhorn   Jonathan W. Uhr

RECENT TITLES

See pages 333 and 334 for previous titles in the series.

Eleventh International
Congress of Anatomy, Part A

GLIAL AND NEURONAL
CELL BIOLOGY

**Proceedings Sponsored by the International Federation of
Associations of Anatomists and the Mexican Society of Anatomy
August 17–23, 1980, Mexico City, Mexico**

Editor-in-Chief
ENRIQUE ACOSTA VIDRIO
President of the National
Organizing Committee
President of the International
Federation of Anatomy

Editor
SERGEY FEDOROFF
Department of Anatomy
University of Saskatchewan
Saskatoon, Canada

1981

ALAN R. LISS, INC. • NEW YORK

Address all Inquiries to the Publisher
Alan R. Liss, Inc., 150 Fifth Avenue, New York, NY 10011

Copyright © 1981 Alan R. Liss, Inc.

Printed in the United States of America.

Library of Congress Cataloging in Publication Data
International Congress of Anatomy (11th: 1980:
  Mexico City, Mexico)
    Eleventh International Congress of Anatomy: pro-
ceedings.

    (Progress in clinical and biological research;
59)
    Includes index.
    Contents: pt. A. Glial and neuronal cell
biology — pt. B. Advances in the morphology of
cells and tissues — pt. C. Biological rhythms in
structure and function.
    1. Neurobiology — Congresses. 2. Neuroanatomy —
Congresses. I. Acosta Vidrio, Enrique. II. Inter-
national Federation of Associations of Anatomists.
III. Mexican Society of Anatomy. IV. Series.
[DNLM: 1. Neuroglia — Congresses. 2. Neurology —
Congresses. W1 PR668E v. 59A / WL 102 G558 1980]
QP351.I76 1980   599.01'88   81-2778
ISBN 0-8451-0059-9 (set)   AACR2

Contents

Contributors

Enrique Acosta Vidrio, President of the National Organizing Committee of the Eighth International Congress of Anatomy and President of the International Federation of Anatomy

Erle K. Adrian, Jr., Department of Anatomy, The University of Texas Health Science Center at San Antonio, San Antonio, Texas **[113]**

J.J. Anders, NINCDS, National Institutes of Health, Bethesda, Maryland 20205 **[21]**

M.A. Barca, Instituto Cajal, Velázquez 144, Madrid 6, Spain **[37]**

H.G. Baumgarten, Department of Neuroanatomy and Electron Microscopy, Free University of Berlin, 1000 Berlin 33, Federal Republic of Germany **[187]**

F. Bigaré, Department of Anatomy, Free University of Brussels V.U.B., Belgium **[259]**

W.F. Blakemore, Department of Clinical Veterinary Medicine, Madingley Road, Cambridge University, Cambridge CB3 OES, United Kingdom **[105]**

M.W. Brightman, NINCDS, National Institutes of Health, Bethesda, Maryland 20205 **[21]**

A. Carrato, Instituto Cajal, Velázquez 144, Madrid 6, Spain **[37]**

Haydée V. Castejón, Unidad de Investigaciones Biológicas, Facultad de Medicina, Universidad del Zulia, Apartado 526, Maracaibo, Venezuela **[249]**

Orlando J. Castejón, Unidad de Investigaciones Biológicas, Facultad de Medicina, Universidad del Zulia, Apartado 526, Maracaibo, Venezuela **[249]**

S. Chen, Department of Physiology and Biophysics, New York University Medical Center, 550 First Avenue, New York, NY 10016 **[229]**

F. Colin, Laboratory of General Physiology, Brussels Free University, Brussels, Belgium **[269]**

Stephen J. DeArmond, Stanford University School of Medicine, Stanford, California 94305 **[65]**

J. DeFelipe, Sección de Neuroanatomía Comparada, Instituto Cajal, CSIC, Madrid 6, Spain **[291]**

Jean C. Desclin, Laboratory of Histology, Brussels Free University, Brussels, Belgium **[269]**

Lawrence F. Eng, Department of Pathology, Veterans Administration Medical Center, Palo Alto, California 94304 **[65]**

A. Fairén, Sección de Neuroanatomía Comparada, Instituto Cajal, CSIC, Madrid 6, Spain **[291]**

S. Fedoroff, Department of Anatomy, University of Saskatchewan, Saskatoon, Canada **[xv, 1]**

The number in bold type following a contributor's affiliation is the opening page number of that contributor's article.

Jean-Francois Foncin, Ecole Pratique des Hautes Etudes and Unite 106, I.N.S.E.R.M. Laboratoire Montyon, La Salpètrière, F75651 Paris, Cedex 13, France [171]

S. Fujita, Department of Pathology, Kyoto Prefectural University of Medicine, Kawaramachi, Kyoto 602, Japan [141]

L.J. Garey, Institute of Anatomy, University of Lausanne, Rue du Bugnon 9, 1011 Lausanne, Switzerland [303]

N.M. Gerrits, Department of Anatomy, University of Leiden, Wassenaarseweg 62, 2333 AL Leiden, The Netherlands [259]

L. Hertz, Department of Pharmacology, University of Saskatchewan, Saskatoon, Saskatchewan S7N OWO, Canada [45]

D.E. Hillman, Department of Physiology and Biophysics, New York University Medical Center, 550 First Avenue, New York, New York 10016 [229]

J.P. Homung, Institute of Anatomy, University of Lausanne, Rue du Bugnon 9, 1011 Lausanne, Switzerland [303]

Kikuko Imamoto, Department of Anatomy, Shiga University of Medical Science, Ohtsu, Shiga 520-21, Japan [125]

D.G. Jones, Department of Anatomy and Human Biology, University of Western Australia, Nedlands, W.A. 6009, Australia [217]

V.I. Kalnins, Department of Anatomy, Division of Histology, University of Toronto, Toronto, Canada [1]

T. Kitamura, Department of Pathology, Kyoto Prefectural University of Medicine, Kawaramachi, Kyoto 602, Japan [141]

L. López-Mascaraque, Sección de Neuroanatomía Comparada, Instituto Cajal, CSIC, Madrid, Spain [281]

J. Manil, Laboratorium voor Fysiologie en Fysiopathologie, Vrije University of Brussels, Brussels, Belgium [269]

E. Marani, Department of Anatomy, University of Leiden, Wassenaarseweg 62, 2333 AL Leiden, The Netherlands [259]

R. Martínez-Ruiz, Sección de Neuroanatomía Comparada, Instituto Cajal, CSIC, Madrid 6, Spain [291]

F. Moritz, Department of Neuroanatomy and Electron Microscopy, Free University of Berlin, 1000 Berlin 33, Federal Republic of Germany [187]

L. Müller, Department of Morphology, Netherlands Ophthalmic Research Institute, P.O. Box 6411, 1005 EK Amsterdam, The Netherlands [199]

J.A. Paterson, Department of Anatomy, University of Manitoba, Winnipeg, Manitoba, Canada [83]

Ch. Pilgrim, Abt. Klinische Morphologie der Universität Ulm, Oberer Eselsberg, D-7900 Ulm, BRD [59]

I. Reisert, Abt. Klinische Morphologie der Universität Ulm, Oberer Eselsberg, D-7900 Ulm, BRD [59]

Alex F. Roche, Fels Research Institute, Department of Pediatrics, Wright State University School of Medicine, Yellow Springs, Ohio [321]

Arnold B. Scheibel, Departments of Anatomy and Psychiatry and Brain Research Institute, UCLA Medical Center, Los Angeles, California [311]

Robert L. Schelper, Department of Pathology, The University of Texas Health Science Center at San Antonio, San Antonio, Texas **[113]**

H.G. Schlossberger, Max-Planck-Institute for Biochemistry, Martinsried, Federal Republic of Germany **[187]**

Robert P. Skoff, Department of Anatomy, Wayne State University School of Medicine, 540 E. Canfield, Detroit, Michigan 48201 **[93]**

L. Subrahmanyan, Department of Anatomy, Division of Histology, University of Toronto, Toronto, Canada **[1]**

A. Toledano, Universidad Complutense, Madrid, Spain **[37]**

Y. Tsuchihashi, Department of Pathology, Kyoto Prefectural University of Medicine, Kawaramachi, Kyoto 602, Japan **[141]**

F. Valverde, Sección de Neuroanatomía Comparada, Instituto Cajal, CSIC, Madrid, Spain **[281]**

J. Voogd, Department of Anatomy, Free University of Brussels V.U.B., Belgium **[259]**

G. Vrensen, Department of Morphology, Netherlands Ophthalmic Research Institute, P.O. Box 6411, 1005 EK Amsterdam, The Netherlands **[199]**

R. White, Department of Anatomy, University of Saskatchewan, Saskatoon, Canada **[1]**

Eleventh International Congress of Anatomy

CONTENTS OF PART B: ADVANCES IN THE MORPHOLOGY OF CELLS AND TISSUES
Miguel A. Galina, *Editor*

SOME FUNCTIONAL AND MORPHOLOGICAL ASPECTS OF HEMATOPOIESIS

MORPHOLOGY OF THE RESPIRATORY SYSTEM

MORPHOLOGY OF THE REPRODUCTIVE SYSTEM

CONTENTS OF PART C: BIOLOGICAL RHYTHMS IN STRUCTURE AND FUNCTION
Heinz von Mayersbach, Lawrence E. Scheving, and John E. Pauly, *Editors*

Preface

The papers in this volume are drawn from six symposia in the field of neurobiology held during the Eleventh International Congress of Anatomy in Mexico City in August 1980. Professor Enrique Acosta Vidrio, President of the Congress, had asked anatomists from many countries to suggest topics for the symposia, and those selected represent areas of rapid advance and wide interest.

Three symposia dealt with the topic Recent Advances in Structure and Function of Glial Cells, suggested by Dr. C. Leblond (Canada): one on Astrocytes was convened by Dr. S. Fedoroff (Canada), one on Oligodendrocytes, by Dr. R.P. Skoff (U.S.A.), and one on Microglia, by Dr. A. Privat (France).

A symposium on Morphological Aspects of Interneuronal Communication was convened by Dr. D.G. Jones (Australia), another, on Morphological Basis of Neurophysiology of the Cerebellum, by Dr. R. Llinas (U.S.A.), and one on Contribution of Metallic Impregnation to Neuroanatomy, by Dr. M. Marin-Padilla (U.S.A.).

Participants in the symposia were a broadly representative international group, coming from 12 countries: Australia, Belgium, Canada, France, Japan, Spain, Switzerland, The Netherlands, United Kingdom, U.S.A., Venezuela, and West Germany.

A unique feature of the Congress and hence of this volume was the organization of a separate symposium on each type of glial cell of the central nervous system, a sign of growing interest in the role of glial cells in the functioning of the nervous system.

I have arranged the papers for publication, including some special lectures presented at the Congress, in seven sections, and in so doing, have taken some liberties. Thus, the contents of each section do not correspond exactly to the program of each symposium. The final paper, on the topic Development of the Brain, was given as a special lecture.

I should also point out that it was the responsibility of each author to submit camera-ready copy; in the interest of speedy publication, some sacrifice of editorial consistency was made.

I would like to thank Dr. M.A. Galina, Coordinator of Scientific Sessions for the Congress, and Sra. Ma. Victoria de Acevedo, Administrative Coordinator, who were extremely helpful in running the symposia and gathering manuscripts. I am grateful also to Dr. F. Oteruelo and Dr. M. Issa for assistance with the translation of some manuscripts, to E. Fedoroff for assistance with the editing, and to I. Karaloff for preparation of manuscripts.

Sergey Fedoroff

STRUCTURE AND FUNCTION
OF ASTROCYTES

Eleventh International Congress of Anatomy:
Glial and Neuronal Cell Biology, pages 1—19
© **1981 Alan R. Liss, Inc., 150 Fifth Avenue, New York, NY 10011**

PROPERTIES OF PUTATIVE ASTROCYTES IN COLONY CULTURES OF MOUSE NEOPALLIUM

S. Fedoroff*, R. White*, L. Subrahmanyan** and
V.I. Kalnins**
*Department of Anatomy, University of Saskatchew-
an, Saskatoon, Canada **Division of Histology,
Department of Anatomy, University of Toronto
Toronto, Canada

Nervous tissue has its embryonic origin in primitive proliferating cells, the ventricular cells. These cells diverge into a number of cell lineages each of which under-goes differentiation into specialized cell types. Tissue culture provides nearly ideal conditions for the study of cell lineages. Cells in primary cultures are direct descen-dants of cells in vivo and provide continuation of the in situ cell lineage (Fedoroff, 1977b). By carefully selecting the stage of development of the embryo and the culturing conditions it is now possible to obtain specific neural cell types including neurons (Wood and Bunge, 1975; Wood, 1976; Varon, 1977), astrocytes (Booher and Sensenbrenner, 1972; Fedoroff, 1977a, 1978; McCarthy and de Vellis, 1980), oligo-dendrocytes (McCarthy and de Vellis, 1980; Szuchet and Stef-enson, 1980), Schwann cells (Wood and Bunge, 1975; Wood, 1976), or neural cells at a specific stage of their lineage (Fedoroff, 1978, 1980).

Colony culture method. In our laboratory we have devel-oped a colony culture method and have used it to study the astrocyte cell lineage (Fedoroff, 1977a, 1978, 1980). We have used embryos from DBA/1J, C_3H/HeJ and Swiss mice as well as chick embryos to isolate the neopallium aseptically after carefully removing the meninges. The hemispheres were then freed of the basal ganglia, olfactory lobes and hippo-campus and divided by means of microscalpels into small fragments which were then dissociated by gently forcing the tissue through sterile "Nitex" ®mesh (pore size 75 μm). The cells were then suspended in a growth medium consisting of Eagle's Minimum Essential Medium (MEM) containing a four-fold concentration of vitamins, a double concentration of amino acids (except glutamine, which was kept at the 2 mM level), 7.5 mM glucose and 5% horse serum (v/v). Cell viability was determined by the Nigrosine dye exclusion technique (Kaltenback et al., 1958). The cells, in various dilutions in a total volume of 2.5 ml growth medium, were plated in 60 mm Falcon petri dishes. The cultures were incubated at 37°C in a humidified atmosphere containing 5% CO_2 in air. After three days of incubation, round, refractile cells could be seen attached to the plastic dish surface and many single cells, cell clumps and cell debris were floating in the medium. At this stage the cell debris and non-attached cells were removed and fresh medium was added. On subsequent culturing the dissociated cells began to proliferate and to form discrete colonies which varied in size, density and overall morphology (Fig. 1). The number of colonies formed depends on the number of viable cells initially plated as well as on the age of the embryo (Fedoroff, 1977a, 1978, 1980).

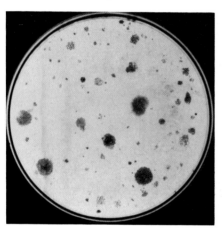

Fig. 1. Culture from dissociated 15-day mouse embryo cerebral hemispheres grown for 14 days in 60 mm Falcon petri dish. Cells form discrete colonies varying in size, density and morphology.

Colony types. Based on morphological criteria six distinct types of colonies have been identified and designated A to F (Fedoroff, 1977a). The frequency of occurrence of the various colony types varies according to the age of the embryo or postnatal mouse, the source of cells in the CNS, duration of culturing and the culture medium used (Fedoroff, 1977a, 1978, 1980; Fedoroff and Hall, 1979; Juurlink et al., 1980). In this paper however, only the relationship between type A colonies and type C colonies will be discussed. Cultures initiated from young embryos formed type A colonies in high frequency and type C colonies in low frequency; whereas cultures initiated from newborn animals formed type C colonies in high frequency and type A colonies in low frequency. Up to seven days after plating incidence of the two colony types was about the same but after seven days the ratio between the two began to change. Also, at seven days, the size of the colonies was such that the various types could be identified easily. For these reasons, 7-day cultures were used to determine the frequency of occurrence of proliferating cell types in neural tissue. We believe that the 7-day colonies still reflect fairly closely the composition of the proliferating cell population removed from the CNS and can, therefore, be used to assay the cell types in this population at any given stage of CNS development. Shifts in the incidence of colony types on further culturing were used to trace cell differentiation or progression along the lineage (Fedoroff, 1979, 1980). For example, 7-day cultures prepared from the neopallium of 14 day old mouse embryos (E14) had a high frequency of type A and a much lower frequency of type C colonies. After 14 days in culture the frequency of type A colonies decreased and that of type C colonies increased (Fedoroff, 1978). These observations were interpreted to mean that type A colonies in cultures give rise to type C colonies (Fedoroff, 1978). This was subsequently confirmed through direct observation of the colonies by time lapse cinemicrography (Fedoroff, 1978). It should be noted that the change in the cell population of the CNS in embryos of increasing age, as assayed by colony cultures, was the same as the change observed when type A colonies were cultured for 3 or 4 weeks (Fedoroff, 1978, 1980). We are therefore convinced that the changes observed in cultures correspond to those occurring in vivo.

Cells of type A colonies. The type A colonies are composed of epithelial-like cells (Fig. 2) and as mentioned, occur in a very high frequency in cultures from younger embryos (Fedoroff, 1978). It does not seem likely that type A colonies originate from fibroblasts, endothelial cells, blood cells or smooth muscle cells, because each of these cell types has a quite different morphological appearance and growth pattern in culture. The most likely source of the cells in type A colonies seems to be the neuroectoderm. The only other derivatives of neuroectoderm with an epithelial-like appearance which might have been present in our cultures are cells of the pia mater. However, when we cultured cells from pia mater, type A colonies did not form (see also Sensenbrenner and Mandel, 1974; Moonen, 1980). We concluded, therefore that cells comprising the type A colonies are not descendants of pia mater, but originated directly from neuroectoderm. Ultrastructural examination of type A colony cells indicated that the cells are indeed very immature. The cells have large oval nuclei with evenly distributed chromatin within which only a few patches of condensed chromatin were observed. The cytoplasm is rich in free ribosomes arranged in polysomes but contains relatively few mitochondria and cisternae of rough endoplasmic reticulum. Inclusion bodies, Golgi complexes, 10 nm filaments and microtubules were also observed in the cytoplasm (Fedoroff, 1980; Juurlink et al., 1980).

The fine structure of type A colony cells thus closely resembles that of the "pale" cells in the subventricular zone of newborn (PO) mice described by Smart (1961), Fisher (1967), Lewis (1968), Blakemore (1969), Blakemore and Jolly (1972), Privat and Fulcrand (1977), Imamoto et al., (1978) and Sturrock and Smart (1980). To confirm that the cells of type A colonies originated from the subventricular zone, the zone was carefully dissected from the rest of the neopallium. The number of colonies and the frequency of the type A colony-forming cells obtained from the subventricular zone and from the rest of the neopallium were then compared by the colony culture assay method (Juurlink et al., 1980). It was found that the subventricular zone of PO mice contributed 73% of all the colonies and 70% of all type A colony forming cells in the neopallium. These observations, together with the fact that the ultrastructure of the "pale" cells of the subventricular zone resembles that of the cells forming type A colonies, strongly suggest that the cells which form type A colonies originate from the subventricular zone of the neopallium.

Cells of type C colonies and formation of putative astrocytes. By observing type A colonies in cultures continuously for four weeks with phase contrast microscopy and time-lapse cinemicrography we noticed that type A colonies transformed into type C colonies. The epithelial-like cells of these colonies were no longer closely apposed to adjacent cells but made contact with them by means of many short slender, interdigitating processes (Fig. 3) (Fedoroff, 1977a, 1978, 1980).

The cells of the "mature" type C colonies (present in cultures of two weeks or more), grown in the presence of dBcAMP, form star-shaped cells which resemble astrocytes (Figs. 4 and 5). If the growth of marked individual type A colonies is followed for a period of four weeks during which dBcAMP is added to the medium for the last two weeks type A colonies are observed to gradually develop into type C colonies and eventually into colonies composed of star-shaped

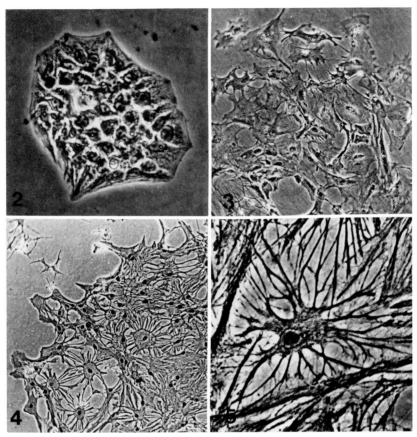

Fig. 2 Type A colony composed of epithelial-like astrocyte progenitor cells. Seven-day culture, phase contrast microscopy. x300.

Fig. 3 Type C colony consisting of cells with many short, slender processes and centrally placed nuclei. Ten-day culture, phase contrast microscopy. x90.

Fig. 4. Colony, consisting of star-shaped putative astrocytes. Culture was grown for first two weeks in normal growth medium and for the last two weeks in medium to which dBcAMP was added. Phase contrast microscopy. x90.

Fig. 5. Putative astrocyte, having many processes with secondary and some tertiary branching from a culture similar to that shown in Fig. 4. Phase contrast microscopy. x420.

astrocytes (Fig. 4). Whether or not cells of type A colonies
are pluripotential, i.e., whether under different environmental conditions they can give rise to cells of lineages
other than the astrocyte lineage, remains to be determined.

     Effect of culture environment on astrocyte differentia-
tion. It is well known that the morphology of cells in culture depends to some extent on the culture environment. To
determine the extent to which cells belonging to the astrocyte cell lineage are affected by different culture conditions
and how the conditions influence the differentiation of these
cells, a number of experiments were undertaken. They showed
that plating the cells on polylysine-coated culture dishes
and dissociation and replating of cells of type A colonies
accelerates transformation of type A into type C colonies.
In contrast, increasing the concentration of horse serum,
which seems to inhibit division, also inhibits the transformation from type A to type C colonies (Fedoroff and Hall,
1979). Moonen et al., (1976) reported that in monolayer
cultures the transformation of rat astrocyte precursor cells
into star-shaped cells, as well as permanency of the transformation, depends on the culture medium used. They found
that growing precursor cells in MEM with fetal calf serum
for ten days, and then treating the cultures with dBcAMP,
slowly induced the cells to transform into star-shaped
astrocyte-like cells which did not change their morphology
appreciably on removal of dBcAMP (Moonen et al., 1975). In
addition, they found that such cells developed bundles of
intermediate filaments in their cytoplasm (Moonen et al.,
1976). Our findings using the culture system are essentially
the same and fully support the observations of Moonen et al.,
(1975, 1976), and of Shapiro (1973) who also observed slow
changes in cell morphology in monolayer cultures of fetal
brain neural cells on addition of mono-butyryl cyclic AMP
(mBcAMP) to cells grown in the presence of serum in Dulbecco's
modified Eagle's medium. The transformed star-shaped cells
in our colonies also develop intermediate size filaments in
their cytoplasm (Fedoroff, 1980; Juurlink et al., 1980) and
do not lose their astrocyte-like appearance on removal of
dBcAMP from the medium. It seems that our culture conditions
arrest the progression of most astrocyte precursors through
the lineage of differentiation at the type C colony level.
In the presence of dBcAMP, however, the cells of type C colonies overcome this obstacle and most of them are now able
to complete progression through their lineage of differentiation and change into large star-shaped putative astrocytes
(Juurlink et al., 1980; Fedoroff, 1980).

Moonen et al. (1975) reported that replacement of the
serum with dBcAMP in cultures of rat astrocyte precursor
cells grown in fetal calf serum supplemented Eagle's basal
medium (BME) rather than MEM for ten days, induced rapid morphological changes leading to the formation of star-shaped
cells. However, this change is not permanent since after
removal of dBcAMP or after addition of serum to the culture
medium the cells reverted to their original morphology.
Essentially similar observations were also made on monolayer
subcultures of cells obtained from fetal rat cerebrums and
cerebellums by Lim et al. (1973) and more recently on monolayer cultures of cells from neonatal rat cerebral hemispheres
by Manthorpe et al. (1979). From these studies on the effect
of the environment on astrocyte differentiation it can be
concluded that only the irreversible changes should be considered as part of the differentiation process in astrocytes,
as suggested by Moonen et al., 1975.

Distribution of cytoskeletal proteins and their precursors.
The colony culture method (Fedoroff, 1977a, 1978, 1980) provides an ideal system in which to study the changes in the
distribution of the different fiber systems during differentiation of astrocytes and how these changes are related to changes
in cell shape. It also allows determination of the time of
appearance of the cytoskeletal proteins specific for glial
cells (Bignami and Dahl, 1977; Schachner et al., 1977; Eng,
1980) during the irreversible transformation of astrocyte
precursor cells into astrocyte-like cells in dBcAMP-treated
cultures. We used indirect immunofluorescence and antibodies
specific to each of the following proteins: a) Glial Fibrillary Acidic Protein (GFAP) (courtesy of Dr. E. Bock); b)
glial filament protein (GFP) recently characterized and shown
to be specific for astrocytes in frozen sections of brain
(V.I. Kalnins et al., manuscript in preparation); c) vimentin
(courtesy of Dr. E. Wang); d) tropomyosin (Jorgensen et al.,
1975); and e) tubulin (Connolly et al., 1977). For immunofluorescence studies, colonies of cells on glass coverslips
from cultures that were treated or untreated with dBcAMP were
fixed with methanol followed by acetone, both at -20°C
(Connolly et al., 1978; Connolly and Kalnins, 1978), before
treatment with the antisera to visualize the distribution of
fiber systems containing GFAP, GFP, vimentin and tubulin. To
visualize the distribution of the tropomyosin-containing micro-
filaments the cultures were fixed in 3.5% paraformaldehyde
and then postfixed in acetone (Lazarides, 1975).

The results showed that virtually all cells from type C
colonies grown for four weeks in culture were positively

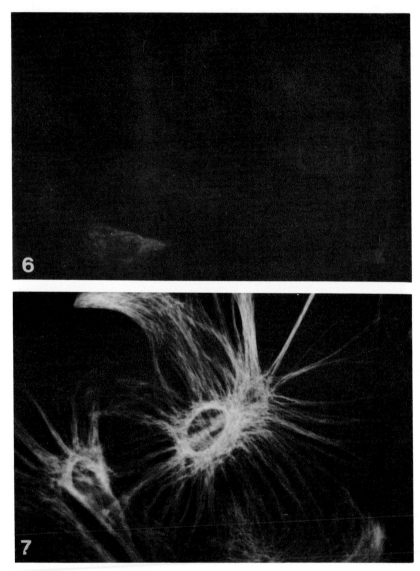

See legends, page 10.

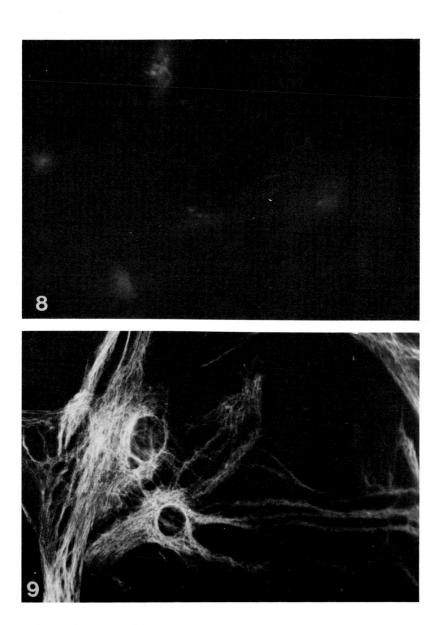

See legends, page 10.

stained with antisera to vimentin (Fig. 10), tropomyosin (Fig. 13 and 14) and tubulin (Fig. 12). The staining patterns observed with each of these antisera were different and characteristic and allowed us to visualize the distribution of vimentin type intermediate filaments, microfilament bundles and microtubules, respectively. In contrast, the great majority of cells in these untreated type C colonies remained unstained with antisera to both GFAP and GFP (Figs. 6 and 8) although a few positive cells were evident in most of the colonies.

When type C colonies (after two weeks in culture) were treated with dBcAMP for two weeks, most cells in these colonies transformed into star-shaped putative astrocytes (Figs. 4 and 5). When these colonies were examined by immunofluorescence all the star-shaped astrocytes were positively stained by antisera to both GFAP (Fig. 7) and GFP (Fig. 9). A positively stained finely fibrillar interlacing network was present throughout the cytoplasm and the fibrillar material extended as compact bundles into the cell processes (Figs. 7 and 9). The pattern of staining observed with antiserum to GFAP protein (Fig. 7) was indistinguishable from

---

Figs. 6 and 7. Immunofluorescence in cells of colonies obtained from dissociated newborn mouse neopallium treated with antiserum to GFAP.

Fig. 6. Cells of a C-type colony grown for four weeks in regular medium without dBcAMP. No cytoplasmic networks of filaments are visible and only a diffuse weak background fluorescence is seen. x590.

Fig. 7. Astrocyte-like cells which appear in colonies to which dBcAMP was added for the final two weeks. Positively stained intermediate filaments are present throughout the cytoplasm. x690.

Figs. 8 and 9. Immunofluorescence in cells of colonies obtained from dissociated newborn mouse neopallium treated with antiserum to GFP.

Fig. 8. Cells of a C-type colony grown for four weeks in regular medium without dBcAMP. No cytoplasmic networks of filaments are visible and only a diffuse weak background fluorescence is seen. x680.

Fig. 9. Astrocyte-like cells which appear in colonies to which dBcAMP was added for the final two weeks. Positively stained intermediate filaments are present throughout the cytoplasm. Their distribution was similar to that visualized with antisera to GFAP shown in Fig. 7. x690.

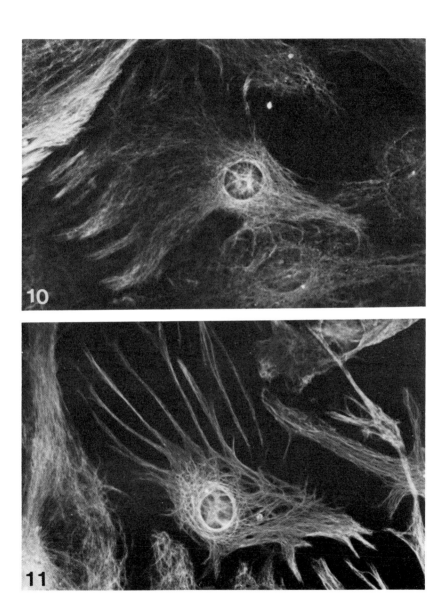

See legends, page 12.

that observed with antiserum to GFP (Fig. 9). As in the
untreated cultures, almost all the cells in these colonies,
including the few that did not transform, were positively
stained by antisera to vimentin (Fig. 11), tubulin and tropomyosin (not shown).

The above results are in agreement with those made recently by Chiu et al. (1980) who found that astrocyte-like
cells in three week old cultures from dissociated forebrains
of one day old rats contained GFAP, actin, and a 58K dalton
protein similar to vimentin.

GFAP, GFP and astrocyte differentiation. The similarity
in the staining patterns observed in our experiments with
antisera to GFAP and GFP, the similarity in the time of
appearance of these proteins during astrocyte precursor cell
transformation and their specificity for differentiated astrocytes are consistent with the suggestion that GFAP, a soluble
protein, and GFP obtained from isolated glial filaments are
similar or identical. Our observation that the appearance
of the glial-specific GFAP and GFP in colony cultures is
related to morphological changes in astrocytes and the observation that the transformed star-shaped cells do not change
appreciably in morphology on removal of dBcAMP from the
medium, support the notion that astrocyte differentiation is
taking place in this culture system. We feel that it is
unlikely that the cells are simply making an adaptive response to culture conditions as suggested by Manthorpe et al.,
(1979).

That a close relationship between the appearance of GFAP
and astrocyte differentiation exists is also supported by
observations made on different brain tumors. Well differentiated astrocytomas, for example, are intensely positive
for GFAP while glioblastomas and astrocytomas of high grade
malignancy are positive only in those areas which contain

Figs. 10 and 11. Immunofluorescence in cells of colonies
obtained from dissociated newborn mouse neopallium treated
with antiserum to vimentin.
Fig. 10. Cells from a C type colony grown for four weeks
in regular medium without dBcAMP have positively stained
vimentin-containing intermediate filaments in the cytoplasm. x730.
Fig. 11. Astrocyte-like cells which appear in colonies to
which dBcAMP was added for the final two weeks, showing
positively stained bundles of vimentin-containing intermediate filaments in the cytoplasm. x660

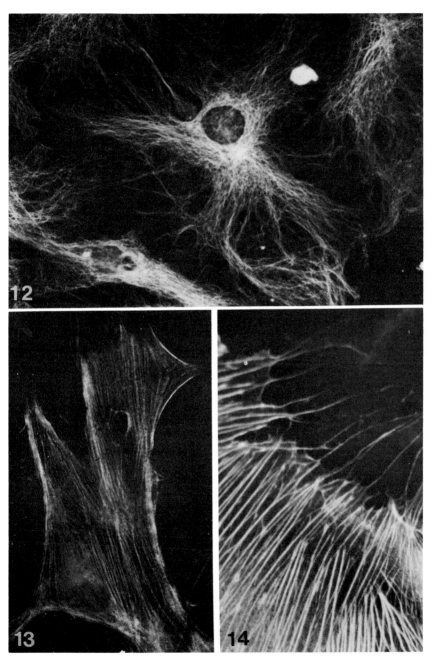

See legends, page 14.

the more differentiated astrocyte (Eng, 1980). Likewise,
cells of medulloblastomas are usually negative for GFAP,
except for positive areas where focal astrocyte differentiation occurs (Deck et al., 1978; Eng and Rubinstein, 1978).

   dBcAMP and astrocyte differentiation. The role of dBcAMP
in astrocyte differentiation is unclear. It seems that dBcAMP
is not an absolute requirement for GFAP synthesis because GFAP
positive cells may also form after removal of serum from the
medium (Moonen et al., 1975; Hertz et al., 1978), or after
addition of a Glial Maturation Factor (Lim et al., 1973,
1977) or brain extracts (Sensenbrenner et al., 1980) to the
cultures. Also, prolonged cultivation (Moonen, 1980; Fedoroff
and Hall, unpublished) may lead to formation of some star-
shaped putative astrocytes that may be GFAP positive even in
cultures to which dBcAMP has not been added. In our colony
cultures which had not been treated with dBcAMP, the relatively few GFAP-positive cells observed tended to have one
or more processes and were morphologically different from
the great majority of cells typically forming the type C
colonies. Therefore it seems that the dBcAMP simply facilitates and accelerates precursor cell transformation into putative astrocytes in serum-containing cultures.

   This is supported by quantitative estimates of GFAP content of monolayer cultures of mouse astrocyte precursor cells.
In these cultures the GFAP content per milligram of protein
was low and constant during the first and second week of culturing; it increased slightly but significantly during the
third week of culturing. However, when dBcAMP was added
during the third week of culturing, this value increased by
a factor of 1.5 or 2.8 depending on whether or not serum was
present in the medium (Hertz et al., 1978; see also Sensenbrenner et al., 1980 and Moonen, 1980).

   Conclusions. The accumulated evidence from a variety
of biochemical (e.g., Hertz, 1977; Hertz et al., 1978;
Schousboe et al., 1980) and morphological (Moonen et al.,
1976; Sensenbrenner, 1977; Cummins and Glover, 1978; Haughen
and Laerum, 1978; Fedoroff, 1978, 1980) studies including the

---

Figs. 12-14. Immunofluorescence in cells of C type colonies
obtained from dissociated newborn mouse neopallium grown in
regular medium without dBcAMP and treated with antiserum to
tubulin (Fig. 12) and tropomyosin (Figs. 13 and 14), showing
the distribution of microtubules (Fig. 12) and tropomyosin-
containing microfilament bundles (Figs. 13 and 14) in the
cytoplasm of these cells. Figs. 12 and 13 x680; Fig. 14
x1100.

present one allow us to conclude that the star-shaped cells observed in cultures of cells from the CNS are astrocytes. However, it remains to be determined whether the accumulation of GFAP and the concomitant changes in cell morphology observed in these cultures resemble astrocyte differentiation or whether they are at least in part, also related to an astrocyte response similar to that which occurs during gliosis in vivo, when reactive astrocytes containing large numbers of intermediate filaments in their cytoplasm are formed (see review by Nathaniel, 1981). It is possible that as the astrocyte precursor cells differentiate in cultures, at one stage they do form cells which closely resemble mature astrocytes in vivo, but that on further culturing these astrocytes then continue to change into cells which resemble reactive astrocytes by increasing in size (Moonen, 1976) and acquiring elevated amounts of GFAP in comparison to normal astrocytes (Bock et al., 1975; Bock et al., 1977).

We anticipate that our colony culture system will help us to understand astrocyte differentiation and to delineate both the sequence of events and the control mechanisms which convert glial progenitor cells into mature astrocytes.

Acknowledgements. This work was done with the support of MRC Grant MT 4235 to S. Fedoroff and MRC Grant MT 3302 to V.I. Kalnins. We are grateful to M. Wassman and O. Kademoglu for the photography and to Irene Karaloff and Brenda Owchar for assistance in preparation of the manuscript.

References

Bignami A, Dahl D (1977). Specificity of the glial fibrillary acidic protein for astroglia. J Histochem 25: 466.

Blakemore WF (1969). The ultrastructure of the subependymal plate in the rat. J Anat 104: 423.

Blakemore WF, Jolly RD (1972). The subependymal plate and associated ependyma in the dog. An ultrastructural study. J Neurocytol 1: 69.

Bock E, Jörgensen OS, Driftmann L and Eng LF (1975). Demonstration of brain specific antigens in short term cultivated rat astroglial cells and in rat synaptosomes. J Neurochem 25: 867.

Bock E, Møller M, Nissen C and Sensenbrenner M (1977). Glial fibrillary acidic protein in primary astroglial cell cultures derived from newborn rat brain. FEBS Lett. 83: 207.

Booher J, Sensenbrenner M (1972). Growth and cultivation of dissociated neurons and glial cells from embryonic chick, rat and human brain in flask cultures. Neurobiology 2: 97.

Chiu FC, Fields KL and Norton WT (1980). Cultured astrocytes contain the 58,000 MW fibroblast filament protein. Trans Am Soc Neurochem 11: 105.

Connolly JA and Kalnins VI (1978). Visualization of centrioles and basal bodies by fluorescent staining with non-immune rabbit sera. J Cell Biol 79: 526.

Connolly JA, Kalnins VI, Cleveland DW and Kirschner MW (1977). Immunofluorescent staining of cytoplasmic and spindle microtubules in mouse fibroblasts with antibody to tau protein. Proc Natl Acad Sci USA 74: 2437.

Connolly JA, Kalnins VI, Cleveland DW and Kirschner MW (1978). Intracellular localization of the high molecular weight microtubule accessory protein by indirect immunofluorescence. J Cell Biol 76: 781.

Cummins CJ and Glover RA (1978). Propagation and histological characterization of a homotypic population of astrocytes derived from neonatal rat brain. J Anat 125: 117.

Deck JHN, Eng LF, Bigbee J and Woodcock SM (1978). The role of glial fibrillary acidic protein in the diagnosis of central nervous system tumors. Acta Neuropathol (Berl) 42: 183.

Eng LF (1980). The glial fibrillary acidic (GFA) protein. In Proteins of the Nervous System. Eds. R Bradhsaw and D Schneider: Raven Press New York p 85.

Eng LF and Rubinstein LJ (1978). Contribution of immunohistochemistry to diagnostic problems of human cerebral tumors. J Histochem Cytochem 26: 513.

Fedoroff S (1977a). Tracing glial cell lineages by colony formation in primary cultures. In Fedoroff S and Hertz L (eds): "Cell, Tissue and Organ Cultures in Neurobiology," New York: Academic Press p 215.

Fedoroff S (1977b). Primary cultures, cell lines and cell strains: Terminology and characteristics. In Fedoroff S and Hertz L (eds): "Cell, Tissue and Organ Cultures in Neurobiology, "New York: Academic Press p 265.

Fedoroff S (1978). The development of glial cells in primary cultures In Schoffeniels E, Franck G, Tower DB, Hertz L (eds): "Dynamic Properties of Glial Cells, "New York: Pergamon Press p 83.

Fedoroff S and Hall C (1979). Effect of horse serum on neural cell differentiation in tissue culture. In Vitro 15: 641.

Fedoroff S (1980). Tracing the astrocyte cell lineage in mouse neopallium in vitro and in vivo. In Giacobini E, Vernadakis A, Shahar A (eds): "Tissue Culture in Neurobiology," New York: Raven Press p 349.

Fisher K (1967). Subependymal zell proliferation und tumor-disposition brachycephaler hunderassen. Acta Neuropathol 8: 242.

Haugen Å and Laerum OD (1978). Induced glial differentiation of fetal and brain cells in culture: An ultrastructural study. Brain Res 150: 225.

Hertz L (1977). Biochemistry of glial cells. In Fedoroff S and Hertz L (eds): "Cell, Tissue and Organ Cultures in Neurobiology," New York: Academic Press p 39.

Hertz L, Bock E and Schousboe A (1978). GFA content, glutamate uptake and activity of glutamate metabolizing enzymes in differentiating mouse astrocytes in primary cultures. Dev Neurosci 1: 226.

Imamoto K, Paterson JA, Leblond CP (1978). Radioautographic investigation of gliogenesis in the corpus callosum of young rats. I. Sequential changes in oligodendrocytes. J Comp Neurol 180: 115.

Jörgensen AO, Subrahmanyan L and Kalnins VI (1975). Localization of tropomyosin in mouse embryo fibroblasts. Amer J Anatomy 142: 519.

Jörgensen AO, Subrahmanyan L, Turbull C and Kalnins VI (1976). Localization of the neurofilament protein in neuroblastoma cells by immunofluorescent staining. Proc Natl Acad Sci USA 73: 3192.

Juurlink BHJ, Fedoroff S, Hall C and Nathaniel EJH (1980). Astrocyte cell lineage. I. Astrocyte progenitor cells in mouse neopallium. J Comp Neurol (in press).

Kaltenback JP, Kaltenback MH and Lyons WB (1958). Nygrosin as a dye for differentiating live and dead ascites cells. Exp Cell Res 15: 112.

Lazarides E (1975). Tropomyosin antibody: the specific localization of tropomyosin in non-muscle cells. J Cell Biol 65: 549.

Lewis PD (1968). The fate of the subependymal cell in the adult rat brain, with a note on the origin of microglia. Brain 91: 721.

Lim R, Mitsunobu K, Li WKP (1973). Maturation stimulating effect of brain extract and dibutyryl cyclic AMP on dissociated embryonic brain cells in culture. Exp Cell Res 79: 243.

Lim R, Turriff DE, Troy SS and Kato T (1977). Differentiation of glioblasts under the influence of glia maturation factor. In Fedoroff S and Hertz L (eds): "Cell, Tissue and Organ Cultures in Neurobiology," New York: Academic Press p 223.

McCarthy KD, de Vellis J (1980). Preparation of separate astroglial and oligodendroglial cell cultures from rat cerebral tissue. J Cell Biol 85: 890.

Manthorpe M, Adler R and Varon S (1979). Development, reactivity and GFA immunofluorescence of astroglia containing monolayer cultures from rat cerebrum. J Neurocytol 8: 605.

Moonen G (1980) Aspects structuraux et fonctionnels de le croissance et de la differenciation d'astrocytes et de neurones cultivés in vivo. Thesis for the degree of d'Agrege de l'Enseignement supérieur, University of Liege.

Moonen G, Cam Y, Sensenbrenner M and Mandal P (1975). Variability of the effects of serum-free medium, dibutyryl-cyclic AMP or theophylline on the morphology of cultured newborn rat astroblasts. Cell Tiss Res 163: 365.

Moonen G, Heinen E and Goesseus G (1976). Comparative ultrastructural study of the effects of serum-free medium and dibutyryl-cyclic AMP on newborn rat astroblasts. Cell Tiss Res 167: 221.

Nathaniel EJN and Nathaniel DR (1981). The reactive astrocyte. In Fedoroff S and Hertz L (eds): "Advances in Cellular Neurobiology" Vol. 2 New York: Academic Press (in press).

Privat A and Fulcrand J (1977). Neuroglia from the subventricular precursor to the mature cell. In Fedoroff S and Hertz L (eds): "Cell, Tissue and Organ Cultures in Neurobiology," New York: Academic Press p 11.

Schachner M, Hedley-White ET, Hsu DW, Schoonmaker G and Bignami A (1977). Ultrastructural localization of glial fibrillary acidic protein in mouse cerebellum by immunoperoxidase labeling. J Cell Biol 75: 67.

Schousboe A, Nissen C, Bock E, Sapirstein VS, Juurlink BHJ and Hertz L (1980). Biochemical development of rodent astrocytes in primary cultures. In Fedoroff S and Hertz L (eds): "Cell, Tissue and Organ Cultures in Neurobiology", New York: Raven Press p 397.

Sensenbrenner M (1977). Dissociated brain cells in primary cultures. In Fedoroff S and Hertz L (eds): "Cell, Tissue and Organ Cultures in Neurobiology", New York: Academic Press p 191.

Sensenbrenner M, Labourdette G, Delaunoy JP, Pettmann B, Devilliers G, Moonen G and Bock E (1980). Morphological and biochemical differentiation of glial cells in primary culture. In Giacobini E, Vernadakis A and Shakar A (eds): "Tissue Culture in Neurobiology", New York: Raven Press p 385.

Sensenbrenner M and Mandel P (1974). Behaviour of neuroblasts in the presence of glial cells, fibroblasts and neuroglial cells in culture. Exp Cell Res 97: 159.

Shapiro DL (1973). Morphological and biochemical alterations in foetal rat brain cells cultured with presence of mono-butyryl cyclic AMP. Nature 241: 203.

Smart IHM (1961). The subependymal layer of the mouse brain and its cell production as shown by radioautography after thymidine-H^3-injection. J Comp Neurol 16: 325.

Sturrock RR and Smart IHM (1980). A morphological study of the mouse subependymal layer from embryonic life to old age. J Anat 130: 391.

Szuchet S and Stefensson K (1980). In vitro behaviour of isolated oligodendrocytes. In Fedoroff S and Hertz L (eds): "Advances in Cellular Neurobiology" Vol I New York: Academic Press p 314.

Varon S (1977). Neural cell isolation and identification. In Fedoroff S and Hertz L (eds): "Cell, Tissue and Organ Cultures in Neurobiology," New York: Academic Press p 237.

Wood PM and Bunge RP (1975). Evidence that sensory axons are mitogenic for Schwann cells. Nature (Lond) 256: 662.

Wood PM (1976). Separation of functional Schwann Cells and Neurons from Normal Peripheral Nerve Tissue. Brain Res 115: 362.

Eleventh International Congress of Anatomy:
Glial and Neuronal Cell Biology, pages 21 – 35
© 1981 Alan R. Liss, Inc., 150 Fifth Avenue, New York, NY 10011

ORTHOGONAL ASSEMBLIES OF INTRAMEMBRANOUS PARTICLES-AN
ATTRIBUTE OF THE ASTROCYTE

J. J. Anders   and M. W. Brightman

NINCDS, National Institutes of Health

Bethesda, MD 20205

Knowledge of the functions performed by astrocytes is
still largely speculative, although it is safe to assume
that some of their activity depends on the structure of their
cell membrane. The large negative potential of astrocytes,
about -70 to -95 mV, seems to be primarily due to K^+ diffusion potentials in vivo (Kuffler & Nicholls, 1966) and
in vitro (Kimelberg et al., 1979). The fluxes of electro-
lytes depend upon a ouabain-sensitive pump associated with
sodium-potassium activated adenosine triphosphatase (Henn
et. al., 1972). Within the parenchyma of the central
nervous system (CNS), they are the cells that are linked
together by a membrane specialization, the gap junction
(Brightman and Reese, 1969) that has come to be regarded
as the route for ionic and metabolic interaction between
adjoined cells (Kuffler and Nicholls, 1976; Gilula, 1977).
The Müller cell of the retina, an astrocytic type of glial
cell, has uptake sites with high affinity for neurotrans-
mitters such as gamma-amino butyric acid (GABA) (Goodchild
and Neal, 1973). Astrocytes also have high affinity sites for
serotonin (Fillion, et al. 1980). It has been suggested that
the uptake of transmitters or potassium ions by glial cells
may be important as a means of terminating their action on
synaptic beds and as a means of cycling carbon-containing
substances between neurons and glia (see Iversen and Kelly,
1975 for cited work).

Figs. 2, 3 and 4. Reactive astrocytes opposite transplanted
superior cervical ganglion (SCG).

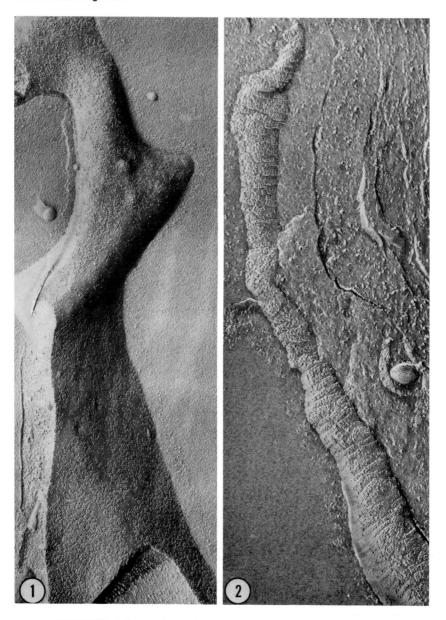

Fig. 1. Marginal astrocyte, jutting into cerebrospinal fluid, is packed with randomly arranged assemblies. X35,000
Fig. 2. Assemblies are highly aligned. X75,000

These properties suggest that the astrocyte cell membrane is involved in a number of activities. We have been attempting to determine whether a function is subserved by a peculiar aggregate of particles residing within the plasma membrane of astrocytes and ependymal cells within the rat brain. These particles can only be displayed by freeze-cleaving the cell membrane and replicating the fractured face with platinum and carbon. When this sort of preparation is then examined by transmission electron microscopy, the P, protoplasmic or inner membrane face is characterized by numerous background particles, about 9-12 nm in diameter, randomly dispersed in an amorphous matrix. Scattered among the background particles, however, are rectilinear or square arrays of small particles or subunits. Each subunit of these orthogonal arrays is 6-7 nm wide (Fig. 1). The aggregates, referred to as assemblies by Landis and Reese (1974), were noted by them to be most numerous in those astrocytes bordering the perivascular and cerebrospinal fluid (CSF).

In order to establish a base line for numbers and distribution of assemblies, so that changes accompanying different functional states can be recognized, fetal, neonatal and adult brain surfaces of rats were fixed in aldehydes and freeze-fractured. The assemblies first appear between the 19th and 20th day of fetal life, an advent that can be regarded as a maturation from astroblast to astrocyte. The number of assemblies increased to reach near-adult levels by the 40th day after birth (Anders and Brightman 1979). The average area of membrane face occupied by the assemblies was also established and found to have increased three to seven fold from fetal to adult stages.

The distribution of assemblies was generally random. Some assemblies tended to form linear patterns, especially those in perivascular astrocytes; most appeared to be randomly scattered. They were most numerous in the superficial layer of the glia limitans. In this subpial layer, they were densely aggregated with areas containing randomly scattered, background particles between the aggregates (Fig. 1). Their number fell off rapidly in successively deeper layers. Square and rectilinear assemblies were interspersed. It is noteworthy, too, that the subunits were confined to the P face and never occupied the E face. On the E face, orthogonal reticules of pits, complementary to the subunit particles, were characteristic (Figs. 3 and 4).

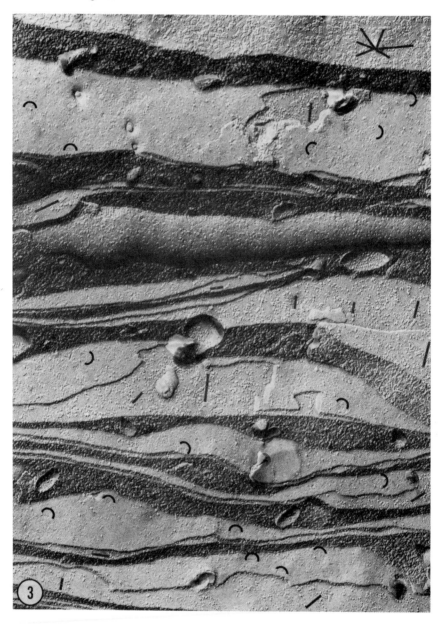

Fig. 3. Assemblies are in all tiers of glial scar. Particles
(lines) on P face, pits (arcs) on E face. X52,000

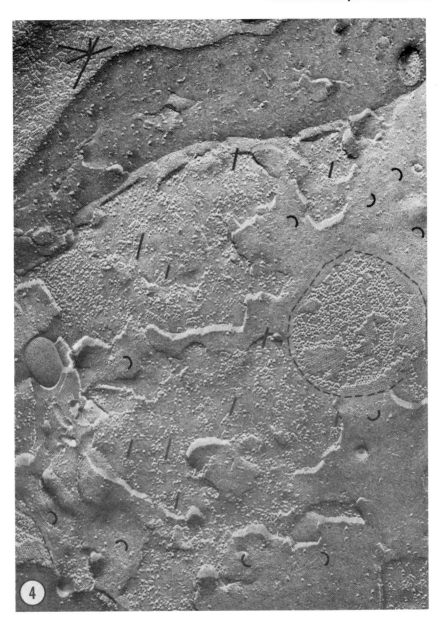

Fig. 4. P face of glial layers contains only assemblies (upper left corner) or assemblies (lines) and gap junction (dashed line). Assembly pits (arcs) are on E face. X72,000

It has been commonly assumed that intramembranous particles are protein, yet particles that are similar in size, have been derived from unilamellar vesicles consisting solely of lipid. When cardiolipin and egg phosphatidyl-choline are mixed to form such single layered vesicles, the vesicles can be made to fuse by the addition of calcium. At the sites of fusion, the freeze-fractured faces contain particles with an average diameter of 10 nm on one face and smaller pits on the opposite one. The particles were re-garded as inverted, lipid micelles sandwiched between two lipid monolayers (Verkleij et al., 1979).

In order to determine whether the assembly subunits were indeed protein in nature, we incubated primary cultures of astrocytes from young rat brains in 10^{-4}M cycloheximide. After three hours of exposure to this inhibitor of protein synthesis, the number of assemblies was markedly diminished (Anders and Brightman 1979). The assembly subunit is not only protein, but one with a high rate of turnover.

The toxicity of drugs such as cycloheximide and the requirements for sustained, known concentration and duration of exposure to various agents made it necessary to use cells maintained in vitro rather than in situ. Because of the regional variation in assembly numbers, the cerebral cortex only was consistently used as the source material. After stripping off the meninges the cerebral cortex and, un-avoidably, the underlying subcortical tissue, was cut away, minced and prepared according to a modification of the Sensenbrenner technique (1977).

Primary cultures of astrocytes, maintained for two to four weeks in vitro, had fewer assemblies in their cell membrane than did cells in situ from rats of comparable age. There was no correlation between cell shape and the content of assemblies. The most common shape of cells grown to confluence was fusiform (Fig. 5). At the periphery of the culture, where the cells were less crowded, they formed branched processes.

Having established the protein nature of assemblies, their average number, size, area, configuration and distri-bution, it was then feasible to determine whether any of these parameters could be modified by different manipulations. One manipulation was that of creating reactive astrocytes,

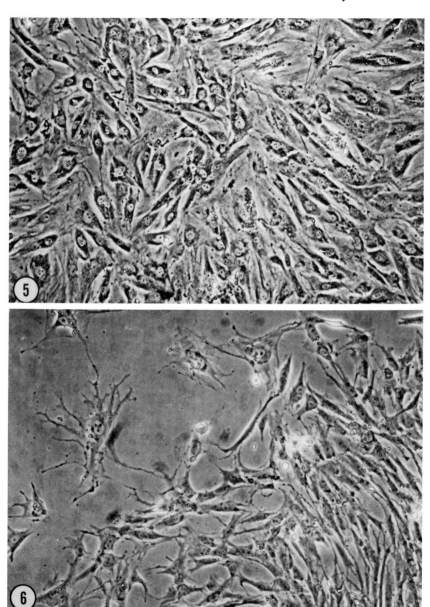

Fig. 5. Astrocyte culture 14 days in vitro. X12.5
Fig. 6. Astrocyte co-cultured with superior cervical
ganglion (SCG). X12.5

the cytological features of which have been well documented (Malamud and Hirano, 1974).

We had found that a discrete gliosis, one confined to a focal region and involving primarily astrocytes with little contribution from fibroblasts or macrophages, could be produced by merely placing a piece of superior cervical ganglion (SCG) on the undisturbed surface of the brain (Rosenstein and Brightman 1978). A few weeks following transplantation of the SCG fragment above the glia limitans, the underlying astrotcytes formed parallel lamellae which, when freeze-fractured, displayed assemblies that were greater in number within all layers, in contrast to the lamellae of a normal glia limitans where the number rapidly diminishes. As illustrated in Fig. 3, the number of assemblies is not only high in the most superficial layer at the top of the photo, but appreciable in deeper layers as well. Some of the alternate layers fractured to reveal the external or E face, contained significant numbers of complementary pits (Fig. 3) of the membrane. The pits are exhibited at higher magnification in another scar where some of the assemblies lie close to gap junctions (Fig. 4). Most assemblies, however, in both normal and reactive astrocytes, are not spatially related to intercellular junctions.

Another striking response of the cell membrane of reactive astrocytes to this SCG stimulus was the conversion from a more or less random distribution of assemblies to a highly ordered one (Anders and Brightman, 1979). The assemblies came into contact with each other, end-to-end, so as to form long trains. The trains themselves were not haphazardly arranged but, rather, lay parallel to one another along the circumference of the glial process. This alignment became established in marginal astrocytes that had either simple (Fig. 2) or plicated excrescences protruding into the CSF (Anders and Brightman, 1979). These parallel rows of assemblies were remarkably organized compared with assemblies on marginal astrocytes that also formed rounded protrusions (Fig. 1). It would appear, therefore, that the orderly alignment of assemblies is not simply due to the curvature of the excrescences. The stimulus provided by the SCG has been the only one, so far, to elicit this change in the distribution of assemblies.

In an attempt to determine whether or not this switch to a highly ordered state might be imposed by some stimulus emanating from the SCG, we have begun co-cultivating primary astrocytes with small fragments of SCG taken from 1 day old rats. A second reason for establishing co-cultures was to see whether neurons "conditioned" the culture medium. It had been noticed that when the primary cultures of astrocytes were fed only on the 3rd and 14th day after plating instead of every few days as prescribed (Sensenbrenner, 1977), the number of assemblies was higher than in those cells fed more frequently. It had also been noted that a few small neurons persisted for at least 14 days in these cultures. The feasibility of neurons as the conditioning source could thus be tested by co-culturing SCG neurons with astrocytes. The method has been to establish the astrocyte growth first (14 days in vitro) either to confluence or to more sparse, patchy colonies and then to add the SCG fragments. The typical shape of astrocytes grown alone and to confluence is fusiform (Fig. 5). The cells at the periphery of a colony of astrocytes emits processes into the surrounding fluid. When freeze-fractured, the fusiform cells were delimited by plasma membranes containing background particles and randomly arranged assemblies like those of astrocytes in situ (Fig. 7).

The explanted fragments of SCG consisted not only of ganglion cells, but of Schwann cells, fibroblasts, macrophages and endothelial cells as well. After 3 days of co-cultivation, some of the cells at the periphery of astrocyte colonies were still fusiform but others had developed radially disposed excrescences, imparting a multipolar shape to the cells (Fig. 6). We have not, as yet, distinguished between the freeze-cleaved membranes of fusiform and stellate cells, but some of the membranes containing assemblies had an unusually large number of oval profiles (Fig. 8). The oval spots resembled the fusion sites of the membrane belonging to pits or caveolae with the plasma membrane of other cell types, such as endothelial.

In addition to changes in the alignment of the assemblies, alterations in their number, distribution, size and shape are possible aftermaths of exposure to various agents. The alterations could be subtle and difficult to recognize. Accordingly, drastic treatment, such as protein denaturation was applied in order to see whether any of these changes could be brought about. Primary cultures of astrocytes were incubated in medium containing 1M and 8M urea for 15 and 30 minutes and in 2M guanidine HCl for 15, 30 and 60 minutes

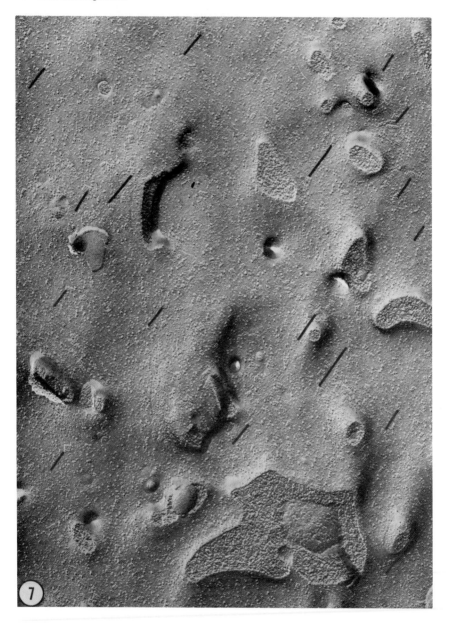

Fig. 7. Cultured astrocytes, like those in Fig. 5, contain assemblies (lines) P face. X60,000

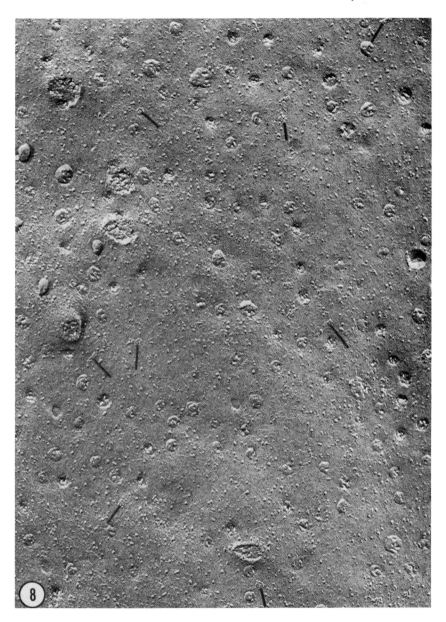

Fig. 8. Astrocytes cultured with SCG contain assemblies (lines) and many oval fusion sites of caveolae with cell membrane. X83,000

respectively. No change in any of the parameters listed above was brought about after exposure to 1M urea.

Thirty minutes after exposure to 8M urea, the cells had disintegrated. Exposure to 2 M guanidine HCl caused a number of reproducible changes. Many of the cells shrunk markedly and had scalloped borders (cf. Figs. 5 and 9). Within their plasma membranes, the background particles became clumped as they do in yeast cells (Necas and Svoboda, 1973) and erythrocyte ghosts (Meyer and Winkelmann 1970) exposed to urea. In the astrocytes, there was not only an aggregation of background particles into separate clumps with bare area between them, but a clumping of assemblies as well (Fig. 10). The aggregation usually appeared to be selective: assembly with assembly without intervening particles, although particles became attached to the periphery of clumped assemblies (Fig. 10). Some of the assemblies were unaltered while others appeared to have lost their alignment. Scattered, small particles, singly or as doublets, suggested some disaggregation of assemblies (Fig. 10). In yeast cell membrane, this total number of background particles did not change but its particles had become redistributed. A striking, grid-like alignment of small particles of the same size was prominent in one of their specimens (Fig. 9, Necas and Svoboda, 1973). This rearrangement may have been an artifact and did not occur within the astrocytic membrane.

The observations on astrocytes in situ and in vitro indicate that the parameters affected by the manipulations used in these experiments are the distribution and number of assemblies. A highly ordered, end-to-end alignment of assemblies is brought about in some reactive astrocytes close to transplanted autonomic ganglion. After the harsh treatment of denaturation, assemblies become clumped in apparently random fashion, and may even disaggregate. The number of assemblies within normal astrocytes in vitro is less than that in situ and still fewer in cultured astrocytes incubated in an inhibitor of protein synthesis. These recognizable changes suggest that comparable alterations may be relatable to other functional states of astrocytes.

This investigation was supported in part by a research grant from the Epilepsy Foundation of America.

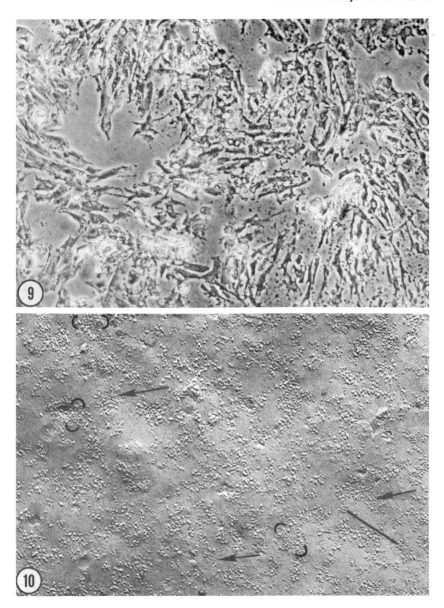

Fig. 9. Astrocytes exposed 30 min. to 2M guanidine. X12.5
Fig. 10. Clumping of background particles and of assemblies
(arcs) after guanidine. Some assemblies are still normal
(lines); others may be disaggreating (arrows). X71,000

REFERENCES

Anders JJ, Brightman MW (1979). Assemblies of particles in the cell membranes of developing, mature and reactive astrocytes. J Neurocytol 8:777-795.

Brightman MW, Reese TS (1969). Junctions between intimately opposed cell membranes in the vertebrate brain. J Cell Biol 40:648-677.

Fillion G, Beaudoin D, Rousselle JC, Jacob J (1980). [^{3}H] 5-HT binding sites and 5-HT-sensitive adenylate cyclase in glial cell membrane fraction. Brain Res 198:361-374.

Gilula NB (1977). Gap junctions and cell communication. In Brinkley BR, Porter KR (eds): "International Cell Biology," New York: Rockefeller University Press, pp 61-69.

Goodchild M, Neal MJ (1973). The uptake of ^{3}H-γ-aminobutyric acid by the retina. Br J Pharmac 47:529-542.

Henn FA, Haljamaë H, Hamburger A (1972). Glial cell function: active control of extracellular K^+ concentration. Brain Res 43:437-443.

Iversen LL, Kelly JS (1975). Uptake and metabolism of γ-aminobutyric acid by neurones and glial cells. Biochem Pharmacol 24:933-938.

Kimelberg HK, Bowman C, Biddlecome S, Bourke RS (1979). Cation transport and membrane potential properties of primary astroglial cultures from neonatal rat brains. Brain Res 177:533-550.

Kuffler SW, Nicholls JG (1966). The physiology of neuroglial cells. Ergebn Physiol 57:1-90.

Kuffler SW, Nicholls JG (1976). "From Neuron to Brain." Sunderland, Massachusetts: Sinauer Assoc.

Landis DMD, Reese TS (1974). Arrays of particles in freeze-fractured astrocytic membranes. J Cell Biol 60:316-320.

Malamud N, Hirano A (1974). "Atlas of Neuropathology." Los Angeles: University of California Press, pp 36-39.

Meyer HW, Winkelmann H (1970). Nachweis der Membranspaltung bei der Gefrierätzpräparation an Erythrozytenghosts und die Beeinflussung der Membranstruktur durch Harnstoff. Protoplasma 70:233-246.

Necas O, Svoboda A (1973). Effect of urea on the plasma membrane particles in yeast cells and protoplasts. Protoplasma 77:453-466.

Rosenstein JM, Brightman MW (1978). Intact cerebral ventricle as a site for tissue transplantation. Nature 275:83-85.

Sensenbrenner M (1977). Dissociated brain cells in primary cultures. In Federoff S, Hertz L (eds): "Cell Tissue and Organ Cultures in Neurobiology," New York: Academic Press, pp 191-213.

Verkleij AJ, Mombers C, Gerritsen WJ, Leunissen-Bijveit L, Cullis PR (1979). Fusion of phospholipid vesicles in association with the appearance of lipidic particles as visualized by freeze-fracturing. Biochimica et Biophysica Acta 555:358-361.

Eleventh International Congress of Anatomy:
Glial and Neuronal Cell Biology, pages 37 – 43
© 1981 Alan R. Liss, Inc., 150 Fifth Avenue, New York, NY 10011

POSTNATAL DEVELOPMENT OF ASTROCYTIC GLIA IN THE CEREBELLUM
OF CYPRINUS CARPIO

Carrato, A., Toledano, A. and Barca, M.A.

Universidad Complutense and Instituto Cajal

Velázquez 144, MADRID-6. Spain

INTRODUCTION

The cerebellar cortex has kept to a basic pattern of
structure throughout evolution. Nevertheless, there are
some particular features within each class (reptilia, birds,
etc.) that can be the result of an adaptative process,
with preservation of the main pattern. In contrast, the
cerebellum has a postnatal development that has no counterpart elsewhere in the central nervous system (CAJAL, 1890).
In the rabbit, the differentiation of the granular layer
from a secondary matrix persists until the second month
after birth; in some teleosts, however, this differentiation continues almost for life (POUWELS, 1978; NIEU-
WENHUYS, 1974). This study analyzes the distribution of
astrocytic glia, both in totally differentiated zones and
in areas with local circuitry in the process of glomerular
neoformation, in 4 to 24 month old Cyprinus carpio
specimens.

MATERIAL AND METHODS
Cerebelli from carp, kindly supplied by the "Junta
de Energía Nuclear" (Madrid), were used. The animals were
anaesthetized by adding EGA's tricaine-methanesulphonate
to the water tank. The skull vault was taken off, ex-
posing the brain and fixing it in situ by flooding with a
solution of 2.5% glutaraldehyde and 5% formaldehyde in
Millonig's buffer. The whole brain was removed, while
under the fixing solution, and 1 cubic mm specimens were obtained from selected sites; they were left in the fixative
for 3 hours at 4°C. Thereafter, tissues were postfixed

with 2% osmium tetroxyde in Millonig's buffer, dehydrated and embedded in Araldite. The sections were studied with a JEOL 100-B electron microscope.

For a previous general orientation, serial sections were obtained from specimens fixed in Carnoy solution and stained with Kiernan's silver method.

RESULTS

I) Astrocytes in differentiated areas

1) Molecular layer. Profuse networks of astrocytic processes surrounding the neuronal fibers of this layer were observed. The thick branches of the Purkinje's dendritic tree became wrapped by glial sheaths of a variable thickness and with a clear cytoplasm (fig. 1). In some cases the sheaths are mostly flattened and develop a multilamellar aggregate. The cytoplasmic organelles are scanty and some mitochondria, smooth endoplasmic reticulum and glycogen granules may be observed. Also the processes of the euridendroid cells are covered by glial sheaths; the cell body of these astrocytes is polymorphic with a big, oval nucleus of granular chromatin, and cytoplasm with gliofibrils, mitochondria, glycogen and smooth endoplasmic reticulum. Bundles of gliofibrils increased markedly from the eighth month of age onward and appear in the soma and processes of astrocytes. Occasionally isolated, stout, glial fibers can be observed running through the field and showing very long and densely packed gliofibrils; they have no apparent relationship to neighbouring dendrites or axons. Some thick pericapillary projections with a high amount of organelles were observed.

Glial sheaths, almost without any organelles, form an envelope around synaptic junctions between parallel fibers and Purkinje dendritic spines. Serial sections demonstrated that the whole structure is often made up of a spine and two eccentrically cap-shaped buttons from a parallel fiber. At this level, the parallel fibers appeared surrounded by astroglial sheets. This accumulation of glial processes interfered with the formation of axon bundles at these levels.

2) Ganglionic layer. At this level, in contrast to mammals, there is not a single layer of cells but a more

complex, irregular stratum, in which Purkinje cells as well as some euridendroid ones are found. The astroglia appear in a smaller proportion than at the molecular layer. The most frequent type related to the ganglionic cells is that of the epithelial glia of Golgi.

3) <u>Granular layer</u>. The astrocytes are not so abundant as in the molecular layer. Their soma is moderate in size and only the vascular processes acquire an important extent and diameter. They also show scant, small bundles of gliofibrils, in a very loose arrangement. The astroglial sheets surround incompletely the cerebellar glomeruli; the most superficial and immature glomeruli offer a more evident glial investment, the deepest and more differentiated glomeruli have a thinner glial covering. Astroglial sheets are also found in relation with the myelinated fibers of this layer.

II) <u>Astrocytes in relation to developing structures</u>

Isolated groups of developing structures, surrounded by astroglial expansions, appear in the most peripheral region of the granular layer, just above the zone where the axonic bundles of granule cells take their origin. Here it is possible to observe branch endings belonging to the developing glomeruli and afferent fibers which, after losing their myelin sheath, soon become wrapped by astrocytic projections (fig. 2), and continue towards the granular cells. These granular cells have descended from the subpial region, from the secondary matrix of the molecular layer (POUWELS, 1978). In fact, these cells have migrated downwards along the ascending axon bundles of some previously matured granule cells; their migration is unrelated to either glial elements or vessels. In their later evolutive stages towards the adult type of granule cell they give off the following types of processes:
a) Stout protrusions with a cytoplasm containing only a few ribosomes. It is on these processes that the mossy fibers progressively develop and differentiate forming serial synapses of a similar pattern to that observed on the Golgi cells in mammals (PALAY, 1965).
b) Thick dendritic processes with abundant organelles, mainly mitochondria, ribosomes and smooth endoplasmic reticulum. These outgrowths lean against mossy fibers and develop two parallel synaptic ribbons, the whole formation being surrounded by astrocytic processes. A diversification

of the dendritic stem and of the mossy endings, as well as
the addition of thick and thin dendrites plus the axonal ends
of Golgi cells constitute the mature glomerulus. During
this progressive evolution the astrocytic investment of the
initial complex becomes relatively smaller until it becomes
almost negligible (figs. 3 and 4).

c) Thin projections containing a cytoplasm endowed
with vesicles of smooth endoplasmic reticulum and a very
slender ending with some neurofilaments. These are fibers
similar to the filopodia described by TENNYSON (1970).
They run among the granule cells and only partially relate
to astrocytes; at times they seem to cross through the glial
sheaths to furnish dendritic terminals to the maturing
glomeruli.

DISCUSSION

Although this study is not concerned specially with
any other glia types, it has been possible to demonstrate
that both the oligodendroglia and the epithelial glia of
Golgi with their Bergmann's fibers show a pattern which,
in our material, does not differ from that observed in the
cerebellum of higher vertebrates. However, the astrocytic
component is of great importance in Cyprinus carpio because
its morphogenetic role persists throughout the whole life,
of the animal, in parallel with the continuous increase of
cerebellar mass and the formation of new granular synaptic
complexes. Similar results have already been shown by
POUWELS (1978) in Salmo gardneri, and, therefore, it seems
possible to suggest that a continuous neurogenesis in postnatal cerebellum may occur also in larger groups of low
vertebrates such as the teleosts.

Our observations on the astroglia in Cyprinus   may be
summarized into two main ideas, as follows:

a) The development and efficient maintenance of a
cover which individualizes and protects the synaptic connections, preventing all contiguity with any other axonal
structures (PETERS and PALAY, 1965); increased complexity
of these systems will further define and isolate other
synaptic compartments (POUWELS, 1978).

b) A subsidiary but important function in the development of new circuits, the astroglia develops concurrently
with other nervous tissue structures. These functional
events of the astroglia may be compared to those described
by ECCLES (1976) in regenerative processes after experi-

mental lesions in the central nervous system of mammals.

REFERENCES

CAJAL, S.R.: A propos de certains éléments bipolaires du
     cervelet avec quelques détails nouveaux sur l'évolu-
tion des fibres cérébelleuses. Intern. Monatschr. Anat.
     Phys., 7/2, 1890.
ECCLES, J.C.: The plasticity of the mammalian central
     nervous system with special reference to new growths
     in response to lesions. Naturwiss., 63, 8-15, 1976.
NIEUWENHUYS, R., POUWELS, E., SMULDERS-KERSTEN, E.: The
     neuronal organization of cerebellar lobe C in the
     mormyrid fish Gnathonemus petersii. Zt.Anat. Entw.
     ges., 144, 315-336, 1974.
PETERS, A., PALAY, S.L.: An electron microscope study of the
     distribution and patterns of astroglial processes in
     the central nervous system. J.Anat., 99, 419 1965.
POUWELS, E.: On the development of the cerebellum of the
     trout Salmo gardneri. V. Neuroglial cells. Anat.
     Embryol., 153, 67-83, 1978.
TENNYSON, V.N.: The fine structure of the developing
     nervous system. In: Development Neurobiology, W.A.
     HIMWHICH ed., 47-116, Springfield, Ch. Thomas, 1970.

EXPLANATION OF FIGURES

1. Dendritic spine of a Purkinje cell with two synaptic
    cup-like endings from a parallel fiber. The whole
    structure is surrounded by several concentric layers
    of astrocytic lamellae.

2. A mossy fiber reaching with its growth cone some
    dendritic buds of a glomerulus at an incipient stage
    of differentiation. Note the large astroglial in-
    vestment.

3. Glomerular complex in a more differentiated stage.
    The external astroglial covering is appreciably re-
    duced.

4. Differentiated area of a glomerulus with numerous syna-
    ptic contacts and no interposition of glia lamellae.

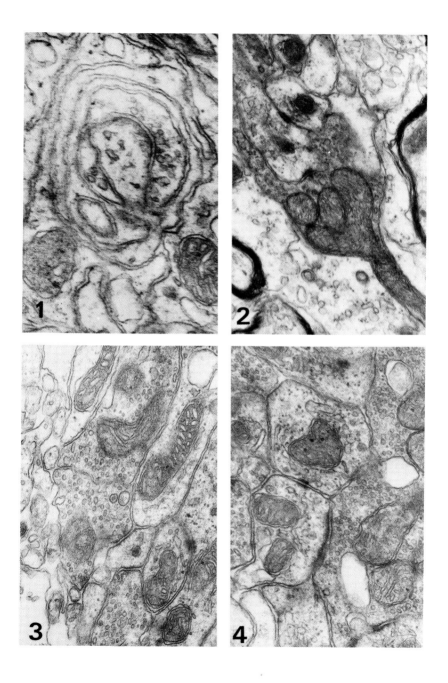

Eleventh International Congress of Anatomy:
Glial and Neuronal Cell Biology, pages 45—58
© 1981 Alan R. Liss, Inc., 150 Fifth Avenue, New York, NY 10011

Functional Interactions Between Astrocytes and Neurons

L. Hertz
Dept. of Pharmacology
University of Saskatchewan
Saskatoon, Saskatchewan
S7N 0W0, Canada

Until recently, it was in general tacitly assumed that biochemical and physiological characteristics of brain tissue reflect events occurring in neuronal cells. This concept was related to the methodologies available since clinical neurological experience, histochemical techniques (e.g., Wallerian degeneration) and neurophysiological experimentation already early had demonstrated the dramatic, longrange consequences of neuronal activity. Glial cells, in contrast, were mainly known to form scar tissue whenever damage had occurred and were regarded as rather inert cells, glueing neurons together.

The first clear demonstration that non-neuronal cells have a major role to play in an important nerve tissue function seems to be that by Geren (1954) that myelin formation in the periphery is a result of an interaction between the axon and the Schwann cell. Modern morphological and cell dynamic techniques have further expanded the knowledge about glial cell functions and characteristics during development, e.g., the guiding role of "radial glia cells" and the severe effect of postnatal undernutrition on glial cell proliferation. Simultaneously, techniques have been introduced which have allowed studies of the biochemistry and physiology of glial cells in the mature nervous system. Such studies have now provided a rather detailed picture of the function of astrocytes. This glial cell type constitutes a large fraction of the volume of the mammalian brain cortex (Pope, 1978); its relative number is especially high in humans and other large, highly developed mammals (Bass et al., 1971); and its surface/volume ratio is very high (Wolff, 1970) due to the presence of a multitude of processes and lamellae (veils), extending from

the astrocytic perikarya and intervening between neuronal cells
as well as between oligodendrocytes and neurons (Palay and
Chan-Palay, 1974). An active role of astrocytes in uptake,
turnover and metabolism of the putative amino acid transmitters,
glutamate and GABA is well established and may obviously modify
neuronal micro-environment. Good evidence is found that
astrocytes also efficiently remove certain other transmitters
(e.g., adenosine) as well as excess potassium from the
extracellular fluid. The effects of, e.g., excess potassium
on astrocytic function might be seen as an automatic answer to
a potassium release from the neurons. Neuronal activity may,
however, determine astrocytic functions also in other ways,
since astrocytes have been found to possess binding sites for
such transmitters as dopamine (Henn et al., 1977), norepinephrine (for review, see van Calker and Hamprecht, 1980), and
serotonin (Hertz et al., 1979a; Fillion et al., 1979) and since
epinephrine or norepinephrine affect nucleic acids in glial
cells in situ (Pevzner, 1965) and energy metabolism in glioma
cell lines (Newburgh and Rosenberg, 1972). These observations
suggest the presence of more specific signals from certain
neurons modifying astrocytic function.

The present paper will describe the astrocytic functions
outlined above and discuss indications suggesting a close

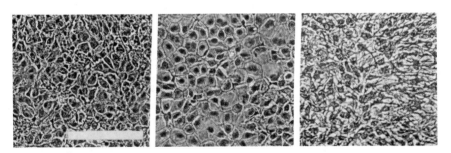

Fig. 1 Phase contrast micrographs of 4-week-old primary
cultures of astrocytes from neonatal mouse brain grown with 20%
fetal calf serum (left), without serum for the last two
weeks (middle) or in the presence of dibutyryl cyclic AMP
(0.25 mM) during the last two weeks (right). These cultures
were fixed with absolute methanol but otherwise treated similarly to those used in the author's experiments. Bar equals
200 μm. Photograph provided by S. Fedoroff.

neuronal-astrocytic interaction in both potassium homeostasis at the cellular level and turnover and metabolism of putative amino acid transmitters. Most of the authors own work in these areas has been carried out using astrocytes in primary cultures obtained from newborn mice. Such cells can be grown in media of different composition, and are shown in Fig. 1 where the homogeneity of the cultures, the absence of fibroblasts or neurons (especially obvious in the cultures grown in the absence of serum), and the astrocytic morphology of the cells after exposure to dibutyryl cyclic AMP should be noted. Corresponding, relatively pure, cultures of cerebral or cerebellar (Messer, 1977) neurons (Fig. 2) can be obtained from the immature mouse or rat brain at certain stages of development (Sensenbrenner, 1977), if neuronal attachment is enhanced by coating of the culture vessels and astrocytic overgrowth is prevented, e.g., by brief exposure to cytosine arabinoside (Dichter, 1978) or culturing in the absence of serum (Yavin and Yavin, 1980). Although some information is available about biochemical characteristics in such cultures (e.g., Hertz et al., 1980; Wood and Hertz, 1980; Yavin and Yavin, 1980) it should be emphasized that their degree of biochemical maturation and "normality" is less well established than that of the corresponding astrocytic cultures. Other preparations in common use include astrocytes and neurons obtained by gradient centrifugation ("bulk-prepared" cells). The characteristics of such cells have been described by, e.g., Hamberger et al. (1975) and Henn (1980).

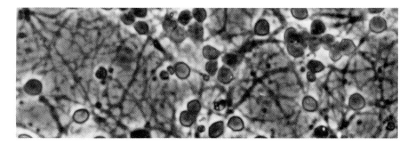

Fig. 2 Culture of cerebellar granule cells from 7-day-old mice after 7 days in culture. Photograph provided by A. Yu.

TURNOVER AND METABOLISM OF PUTATIVE TRANSMITTERS

A simplified diagram of intermediary metabolism in nerve endings and in astrocytes and its relation to the formation and degradation of glutamate and GABA is shown in Fig. 3. These two amino acids are formed in neurons and released in rather large amounts to the extracellular space, at least partly serving a transmitter function. Evidence from work on "metabolic compartmentation" in the intact brain had already suggested that GABA is transferred from its production site to a different cellular or subcellular localization (i.e., possibly glial cells) for subsequent degradation, when it was shown by several different authors that bulk-prepared astrocytes and astrocytoma cells are able to accumulate radioactive GABA and glutamate (for details and references, see, e.g., Hertz, 1979b). Since glutamate (glu in Fig. 3) and GABA are formed from α-ketoglutarate (α-ket in Fig. 3), an intermediate in the tricarboxylic acid (TCA) cycle, this means a loss of TCA constituents from neurons to astrocytes, and Benjamin and Quastel (1975) have suggested that a flow of glutamine (glu NH_2 in Fig. 3), which is formed in astrocytes from glutamate, released to the extracellular space, and taken up by neurons, may be able to compensate quantitatively for this loss (Fig. 3). This suggestion was based upon indirect evidence from experiments on brain slices and, ultimately, the concept of such a glutamate (GABA)-glutamine cycle must be proven or refuted on the basis of direct observations on isolated astrocytes and neurons.

Experiments on astrocytes in primary cultures have confirmed the accumulation of glutamate and GABA into astrocytes and shown that this is a net uptake, not a homoexchange (e.g., the exchange between intracellular and extracellular GABA observed in certain other preparations); they have given the quantitative information that the uptake of glutamate is extremely intense, compared both to the rate of release from neurons and to metabolic rates, whereas the uptake of GABA is considerably less intense and seems to occur into both neuronal constituents and astrocytes (Hertz, 1979b; Hertz and Schousboe, 1980). This quantitative distinction between the two amino acids is supported by the autoradiographic demonstration by McLennan (1976), that glutamate uptake in vivo almost exclusively takes place into glial cells, whereas GABA is accumulated into both astrocytes and neurons (for references, see Hertz, 1979b). The experiments have also demonstrated high activities in astrocytes of the enzymes involved in the subsequent metabolic transformation of GABA and glutamate, including synthesis of glutamine; a preferential localization of glutamine synthetase activity to astrocytes has simultaneously been observed in vivo by Norenberg and Martinez-Hernandez (1979). This is in excellent agreement with the concept that large amounts of glutamate

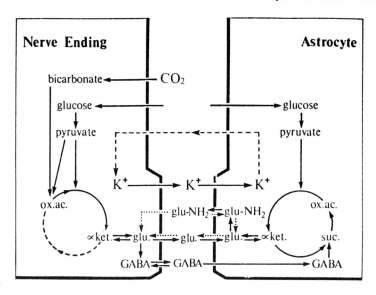

Fig. 3 Diagram of intermediary metabolism and its relation
to the formation and degradation of glutamate (glu) and GABA
in nerve endings or astrocytes. The two circles indicate TCA
cycles, involved in the formation of glutamate and GABA (in
neurons) and the metabolic conversion of these compounds (in
astrocytes?). Fully drawn lines indicate processes which seem
to occur at substantial intensities (for details, see Hertz,
1979b). The Fig. also shows that potassium ions (K+), released
from neurons during activity, seem to be accumulated into
astrocytes. The way of return to the neurons (dashed line) is
unknown.

are transferred from neurons to astrocytes during brain function
and to a considerable extent may be converted to glutamine. The
last step of the suggested glutamate-glutamine cycle, i.e., a
flow of glutamine from astrocytes back to neurons is, however,
not supported by studies of isolated cells, which have demonstrated the complete absence of a high affinity uptake of
glutamine in several different neuronal preparations, including
both cultured cortical neurons and bulk-prepared neurons; in
all these preparations there is a quite intense low-affinity
uptake (Hertz et al.,1980), which might be efficient on account
of a rather high extracellular glutamine concentration in brain

(0.5 mM), <u>but a similar low affinity uptake of glutamine into astrocytes is equally intense</u> (Hertz <u>et al</u>., 1980). There is, therefore, no indications of a preferential glutamine uptake into neurons which must suggest that a net loss of TCA constituents from nerve endings could occur during brain function.

Conceptually, a neuronal loss of TCA constituents could be compensated for by <u>de novo</u> synthesis of oxaloacetate (ox. ac. in Fig. 3) from glucose and CO_2 (Fig. 3). Such a CO_2 fixation is quite intense in brain (Waelsch <u>et al</u>., 1964) and the ultimate consequence of a substantial net transfer of glutamate (and perhaps also GABA) from nerve endings to astrocytes would be that nerve endings synthesize transmitters like glutamate and GABA, <u>but are not able to carry out a complete TCA cycle</u>. This would be in good agreement with the histochemical findings by Kerpel-Fronius and Hajos (1971) that α-ketoglutarate and succinate dehydrogenase activity may be absent in synaptic mitochondria (dashed part of neuronal TCA cycle from α-ket to ox.ac. in Fig. 3). In that case, the main part of the energy production in a metabolic neuronal-astrocytic unit, linked together by a net transfer of glutamate, might take place in astrocytes. A close metabolic interaction between neurons and glial cells has previously been suggested by Hydén (1967) and by Newburgh and Rosenberg (1973), and a substantial amount of evidence for the hypothesis of a neuronal-astrocytic metabolic unit involving a glutamate transfer has been presented by Hertz (1979b).

While uptake of GABA and glutamate into astrocytes has been studied in much more detail than that of other transmitters or putative transmitters, the astrocytic uptake is <u>not</u> limited to these amino acids. Thus, adenosine is taken up both into astrocytes in primary cultures (Hertz, 1978a) and glial cell lines (Lewin and Bleck, 1979); the subsequent fate of this compound is unknown, but it might be as complex as that of glutamate or GABA. Norepinephrine and serotonin have been found to be taken up into bulk-prepared glial cells or glial cell lines (Henn and Hamberger, 1971; Suddith <u>et al</u>., 1978), although the uptake is less intense than that into synaptosomes and preliminary experiments have failed to show a concentrative serotonin uptake into astrocytes in primary cultures (L. Hertz and A. Schousboe, unpublished results).

POTASSIUM HOMEOSTASIS AT THE CELLULAR LEVEL

Whereas glutamate after accumulation into astrocytes can

be converted to glutamine or other metabolites, potassium ions (K+) obviously remain potassium ions. It is, therefore, remarkable that a neuronal-astrocytic interaction also may take place in the case of potassium (Fig. 3).

The first similarity is that potassium, like glutamate, is released from excited neurons to the extracellular space of the central nervous system leading to a measurable increase in potassium concentration during physiological activity (e.g., from the "resting" level of 3.0 to about 4.0 mM), a larger increase (up to about 12 mM) during seizures, and an enormous, completely reversible increase (up to 50-80 mM) during spreading depression or brief exposure to anoxia (for references, see Somjen, 1975; Hertz, 1977). These increases of extracellular potassium concentrations have all been measured in vivo by different groups of neurophysiologists utilizing potassium sensitive micro-electrodes; the in vivo measurements have also convincingly demonstrated that the subsequent reduction to a normal (or in some cases even subnormal) level of potassium in the mammalian central nervous system predominantly is brought about by active, energy requiring re-accumulation into adjacent cells (Vern et al., 1977; Cordingley and Somjen, 1978). Ultimately, potassium ions which originally were released from neurons must obviously be re-accumulated into neurons in order not to deplete these cells for potassium. Since the relative alterations of the extracellular potassium concentrations in the narrow extracellular clefts must be much more pronounced than in the neurons, a re-establishment of a normal extracellular potassium concentration will, however, be more urgent than a correction of the probably rather small decrease in intracellular potassium content in the neurons.

Based upon a glial, and more specifically astrocytic localization of the increase in rate of oxygen uptake by brain tissue in vitro during exposure to high concentrations of potassium (Hertz and Hertz, 1979), it has been suggested that excess extracellular potassium initially is removed by accumulation into astrocytes (for references, see Hertz, 1977, 1979a). More direct support for the concept of such an active potassium uptake into astrocytes (Fig. 3), which is further enhanced when the extracellular potassium concentration is increased above its normal level, has been obtained by the demonstration of an intense net (Hertz, 1979a) uptake of potassium into cultured astrocytes with a K_m of 13 mM (Hertz, 1978b). This uptake is so intense that it would be able to account for the measured rates of removal of excess potassium from the extracellular space in brain cortex in vivo, provided astrocytes in situ have similar characteristics and account for 1/3-1/4 of the total cortical volume.

The further fate of the potassium ions after an initial uptake into astrocytes is unknown. Are they transported via predetermined astrocytic pathways and then released to the extracellular space at another site (Hertz, 1965)? Are they possibly transferred directly from astrocytes to neurons? Does the alleged neuronal uptake occur at another location than nerve endings and are potassium ions subsequently redistributed within neurons (Knull and Wells, 1975)? These questions are gradually becoming accessible for direct experimentation. Evidence has been obtained by Latzkovits, Sensenbrenner and Mandel (1974) that a direct transfer of potassium ions between neurons and astrocytes does occur in mixed neuronal-astrocytic cultures obtained from the chick brain, and Gardner-Medwin (1977) has shown that a transcellular transport of potassium probably occurs in the mammalian brain in vivo. Along the same lines, H. Martins-Ferreira and L. Hertz have in preliminary studies found reversible increases in light scattering in pure cultures of astrocytes. These increases can be induced by certain osmotic alterations in the medium, e.g., the addition of a small amount of concentrated KCl solution, but addition of a corresponding amount of sucrose has much less effect. The alterations of light scattering partly resemble those which have been described during spreading depression in the isolated retina (Martins-Ferreira et al., 1966) and, in this preparation, reflect the passage of a wave of an increase in extracellular potassium concentration (H. Martins-Ferreira and G. Oliveira Castro, personal communication).

NEURONAL SIGNALING TO ASTROCYTES

Uptake into astrocytes of potassium ions or transmitters which have been released from excited neurons, represents one facet of neuronal-astrocytic interactions. A different aspect is that transmitters may serve as specific signals which can modify astrocytic function. This fascinating possibility was under-scored when Henn et al. (1977) demonstrated that bulk-prepared astrocytes have a higher density of high affinity binding sites for dopamine than do synaptosomes, and that the clinical efficacy of antipsychotic drugs was better correlated with their ability to displace dopamine from its astrocytic binding sites than with their ability to displace the transmitter from its synaptosomal binding sites. A substantial amount of information, recently reviewed by Van Calker and Hamprecht (1980), suggests receptor sites on astrocytes not only for dopamine but also for several other transmitters and the interaction of certain of these transmitters with adenylyl cyclase activity. On account of indications of an involvement of β-adrenergic receptors in manic-depressive illness, it may be of special interest that dihydroalprenolol, a β-adrenergic ligand, binds in large amounts to astrocytes in primary cultures and is displaced by all groups of antidepressants tested but not by antipsychotics or anti-anxiety drugs (L. Hertz, S. Mukerji, E. Hertz and J.S. Richardson, submitted for publication); the antidepressants, in turn, counteract an isoproterenol-induced increase in astrocytic production of cyclic AMP (L. Hertz, J.S. Richardson and S. Mukerji, Can J Physiol Pharmacol in press). The events secondary to receptor activation in astrocytes, and thus also the ways in which neuroactive drugs may influence neuronal-astrocytic interactions, are largely unknown (Van Calker and Hamprecht, 1980). One exception to this may be that diazepam (Valium), which binds in large amounts to bulk-prepared astrocytes (Henn and Henke, 1978) and to astrocytes in primary cultures (Hertz and Mukerji, 1980), inhibits uptake of adenosine into astrocytes (Hertz et al., 1979b). This may contribute to the prolongation of adenosine inhibition in vivo which may be causally related to the mechanism of action for the benzodiaze-pines (Phillis et al., 1980).

A considerable amount of evidence suggests that transmitter compounds play a role in growth and differentiation of nervous tissue (e.g., Vernadakis and Gibson, 1974). Since astrocytes possess binding sites for transmitters, this action may be exerted not only on neurons but also on astrocytes. The morphological differentiation of astrocytes which is evoked by culturing with dibutyryl cyclic AMP (Fig. 1) might mimic such a transmitter action since dibutyryl cyclic AMP (dBcAMP) causes an increase in the intracellular level of cyclic AMP in astrocytes in primary cultures (L. Hertz and A. Schousboe, unpublished results), and since prolonged exposure to norepinephrine may lead to a morphological differentiation of astrocytes (Narumi et al., 1978). It is therefore of interest to know to what extent culturing with dBcAMP affects the biochemical characteristics of astrocytes in primary cultures. Although many parameters are affected, most of the alterations are relatively modest (Schousboe et al., 1980). However, the carbonic anhydrase activity shows a very substantial rise (Schousboe et al., 1980), distinct alterations occur in protein synthesis (F.P. White and L. Hertz, Neurochem Res, in press) and the isoproterenol-induced stimulation of adenylyl cyclase activity is almost abolished. The latter phenomenon has been observed both by ourselves (Table I) and Ciesielski-Treska and Ulrich (1980). It seems, however, to represent an abnormal development, maybe caused by continuous, rather than intermittent, exposure to an increased level of cyclic AMP.

Table I

Cyclic AMP, pmol/mg protein

	No dBcAMP during culturing	0.25 mM dBcAMP during culturing
control	93.8±15.6 (9)	54.1± 5.4 (9)
isoproterenol, 1 µM	803.5±82.4 (7)	103.5±25.4 (7)

Production of cyclic AMP by astrocytes in primary cultures incubated with or without isoproterenol for 10 min in the presence of 0.5 mM IBMX, a phosphodiesterase inhibitor (unpublished results by L. Hertz and A. Schousboe).

CONCLUDING REMARKS

In this review it has been attempted to demonstrate that compounds released from excited neurons affect the behavior of astrocytes, which in turn may modify the extracellular concentrations of neuroactive compounds and thus neuronal excitability. Such neuronal-astrocytic interactions are now accessible for experimental investigations, using preparations of isolated neurons and/or astrocytes. During the coming years such studies can be expected to reveal much more details about the role of neuronal-astrocytic interactions under normal and abnormal conditions and both in the mature nervous system and during development.

REFERENCES

Bass NH, Hess A, Pope A, Thalheimer C (1971). Quantitative cytoarchitectonic distribution of neurons, glia, and DNA in rat cerebral cortex. J Comp Neurol 143:481.
Benjamin AM, Quastel JH (1975). Metabolism of amino acids and ammonia in rat brain cortex slices in vitro: A possible role of ammonia in brain function. J Neurochem 25:197.

Ciesielski-Treska J, Ulrich G (1980). Beta adrenergic receptor sensitivity of glial cells in culture. Abstracts, 1st Meeting Internat. Soc. Develop. Neurosci., p. 285.

Cordingley GE, Somjen GG (1978). The clearing of excess potassium from extracellular space in spinal cord and cerebral cortex. Brain Res 151:291.

Dichter MA (1978). Rat cortical neurons in cell culture: Culture methods, cell morphology, electrophysiology, and synapse formation. Brain Res 149:279.

Fillion G, Beaudoin D, Rousselle JC, Fillion MP, Jacob, J (1977). Differences between the serotoninergic receptors present in the synaptosomal and in the glial membranes. Abstracts, 7th Meeting Internat Soc Neurochem, Jerusalem.p. 327.

Gardner-Medwin, AR (1977). The migration of potassium produced by electric current through brain tissue. J Physiol (Lond) 32P-33P.

Geren BB (1954). The formation from the Schwann cell surface of myelin in the peripheral nerves of chick embryos. Exp Cell Res 7:558.

Hamberger A, Hansson HA, Sellström Å (1975). Scanning and transmission electron microscopy on bulk prepared neuronal and glial cells. Exp Cell Res 92:1.

Henn FA (1980). Separation of neuronal and glial cells and subcellular constituents. In Fedoroff S, Hertz L (eds): "Advances in Cellular Neurobiology," New York: Academic Press, p 373.

Henn FA, Anderson DJ, Sellström Å (1977). Possible relationship between glial cells, dopamine and the effects of anti-psychotic drugs. Nature (London) 266:637.

Henn FA, Hamberger A (1971). Glial cell function: uptake of transmitter substances. Proc Nat Acad Sci 68:2686.

Henn FA, Henke DJ (1978). Cellular localization of [^{3}H]-diazepam receptors. Neuropharmacology 17:985.

Hertz E, Hertz L (1979). Polarographic measurement of oxygen uptake by astrocytes in primary cultures using the tissue culture flask as the respirometer chamber. In Vitro 15:429.

Hertz L (1965). Possible role of neuroglia: a potassium-mediated neuronal-neuroglial-neuronal impulse transmission system. Nature (London) 206:1091.

Hertz L (1977). Drug-induced alterations of ion distribution at the cellular level of the central nervous system. Pharmacol Rev 29:35.

Hertz L (1978a). Kinetics of adenosine uptake into astrocytes. J Neurochem 31:55.

Hertz L (1978b). An intense potassium uptake into astrocytes, its further enhancement by high concentrations of potassium, and its possible involvement in potassium homeostasis at the cellular level. Brain Res 145:202.

Hertz L (1979a). Inhibition by barbiturates of an intense net uptake of potassium into astrocytes. Neuropharmacol 18:629.

Hertz L (1979b). Functional interactions between neurons and astrocytes. I. Turnover and metabolism of putative amino acid transmitters. Progr Neurobiol 13:277.

Hertz L, Baldwin F, Schousboe, A (1979a). Serotonin receptors on astrocytes in primary cultures: effects of methysergide, and fluoxetine. Can J Physiol Pharmacol 57:223.

Hertz L, Mukerji S (1980). Diazepam receptors on mouse astrocytes in primary cultures: displacement by pharmacologically active concentrations of benzodiazepines or barbiturates. Can J Physiol Pharmacol 58:217.

Hertz L, Schousboe A (1980). Interactions between neurons and astrocytes in the turnover of GABA and glutamate. Brain Res Bull Suppl 2, in press.

Hertz L, Wu PH, Phillis JW (1979b). Benzodiazepines and purinergic depression of central neurons. Abstract Soc Neurosci 5:404.

Hertz L, Yu A, Svenneby G, Kvamme E, Fosmark H, Schousboe A (1980). Absence of preferential uptake of glutamine into neurons - An indication of a net transfer of TCA constituents from nerve endings to astrocytes? Neurosci Lett 16:103.

Hydén H (1967). Dynamic aspects on the neuron-glia relationship. A study with micro-chemical methods. In Hydén H (ed): "The Neuron," Amsterdam: Elsevier, p. 179.

Kerpel-Fronius S, Hajos F (1971). Attempt at structural identification of metabolic compartmentation of neural tissue based on electron histochemically demonstrable differences of mitochondria. Neurobiol 1:17.

Knull HR, Wells WW (1975). Axonal transport of cations in the chick optic system. Brain Res 100:121.

Latzkovits L, Sensenbrenner M, Mandel P (1974). Tracer kinetic model analysis of potassium uptake by dissociated nerve cell cultures: Glial-neuronal interrelationship. J Neurochem 23:193.

Lewin E, Bleck V (1979). Uptake and release of adenosine by cultured astrocytoma cells. J Neurochem 33:365.

Martins-Ferreira H, Oliveira Castro G de (1966). Light scattering changes accompanying spreading depression in isolated retina. J Neurophysiol 29:715.

McLennan H (1976). The autoradiographic localization of L-[^{3}H] glutamate in rat brain tissue. Brain Res 115:139.

Messer A (1977). The maintenance and identification of mouse cerebellar granule cells in monolayer cultures. Brain Res 130:1.

Narumi S, Kimelberg HK, Bourke RS (1978). Effects of norepinephrine on the morphology and some enzyme activities of primary monolayer cultures from rat brain. J Neurochem 31:1479.

Newburgh RW, Rosenberg RN (1972). Effect of norepinephrine on glucose metabolism in glioblastoma and neuroblastoma cells in cell culture. Proc Natl Acad Sci USA 69:1677.

Newburgh RW, Rosenberg RN (1973). Glucose metabolism in mixed glioblastoma and neuroblastoma cultures. Biochem Biophys Res Comm 52:614.

Norenberg MD, Martinez-Hernandez A (1979). Fine structural localization of glutamine synthetase in astrocytes of rat brain. Brain Res 161:303.

Palay S, Chan-Palay V (1974). Cerebellar cortex: cytology and organization. Springer, New York.

Pevzner LZ (1965). Topochemical aspects of nucleic acid and protein metabolism within the neuron-neuroglia unit of the superior cervical ganglion. J Neurochem 12:993.

Phillis JW, Bender AS, Wu PH (1980). Benzodiazepines inhibit adenosine uptake into rat brain synaptosomes. Brain Res 195:494.

Pope A (1978). Neuroglia: quantitative aspects. In Schoffeniels E, Franck G, Hertz L, Tower DB (eds): "Dynamic Properties of Glia Cells," Oxford: Pergamon Press, p 13.

Schousboe A, Nissen C, Bock E, Sapirstein V, Juurlink BHJ, Hertz L (1980). Biochemical development of rodent astrocytes in primary cultures. In Giacobini E, Vernadakis A, Shahar A (eds): "Tissue Culture in Neurobiology", New York: Raven Press, p 397.

Sensenbrenner M (1977). Dissociated brain cells in primary cultures. In Fedoroff S, Hertz L (eds): "Cell, Tissue and Organ Cultures in Neurobiology," New York: Academic Press, p 191.

Somjen GG (1975). Electrophysiology of neuroglia. Annu Rev Physiol 37:163.

Suddith RL, Hutchison HT, Haber B (1978). Uptake of biogenic amines by glial cells in culture I. A neuronal-like transport system for serotonin. Life Sciences 22:2179.

Van Calker D, Hamprecht B (1980). Effects of neurohormones on glial cells. In Fedoroff S, Hertz L (eds): "Advances in Cellular Neurobiology," New York: Academic Press, p 33.

Vern BA, Schuette WH, Thibault LE (1977). K^+ clearance in
cortex: a new analytical model. J Neurophysiol 40:1015.
Vernadakis A, Gibson DA (1974). Role of neurotransmitter
substances in neural growth. In Dancis J, Hwang JC (eds):
"Perinatal Pharmacology," New York: Raven Press, p 65.
Waelsch H, Berl S, Rossi CA, Clarke DD, Purpura DP (1964).
Quantitative aspects of CO_2 fixation in mammalian brain in
vivo. J Neurochem 11:717.
Wolff JR (1970). The astrocytes as link between capillary and
nerve cell. Triangle 9:153.
Wood JD, Hertz L (1980). Ketamine-induced changes in the GABA
system of mouse brain. Neuropharmacol 19:805.
Yavin E, Yavin L (1980). Sources of choline for developing
cerebral cells. In Giacobini E, Vernadakis A, Shahar A (eds):
"Tissue Culture in Neurobiology," New York: Raven Press,
p 277.

ACKNOWLEDGEMENT

The author's own work has been supported by the MRC
of Canada (Grant #MT5957).

Eleventh International Congress of Anatomy:
Glial and Neuronal Cell Biology, pages 59 — 64
© **1981 Alan R. Liss, Inc., 150 Fifth Avenue, New York, NY 10011**

THE GLIAL CELL AS A MAJOR SITE OF GLYCOCONJUGATE SYNTHESIS
IN THE BRAIN

Ch. Pilgrim and I. Reisert

Abt. Klinische Morphologie
der Universität Ulm
Oberer Eselsberg
D-7900 Ulm, BRD

Biochemical and autoradiographic investigations on the synthesis and transport of glycoproteins in the hypothalamo-
neurohypophysial system of the rat led us to the impression
that glial cells of the hypothalamus may be considerably
more active in this respect than neurons (Pilgrim and Wagner,
1975). We have since tried to systematically investigate this
phenomenon by quantitative electron microscopic autoradiography using several radioactive precursors of glycoconjugate and protein synthesis.

L-(^{3}H)fucose, N-(^{3}H)acetyl-D-mannosamine and L-(^{3}H)
leucine were stereotaxically injected into the ventricular
system of rats. In the case of (^{3}H)fucose, the experimental
times varied between 10 min and 7 days. With the other precursors, the animals survived 30 min. The upper body half
was fixed by vascular perfusion of a formaldehyde/glutaral-
dehyde mixture. Several brain regions were excised, post-
fixed in OsO_4, embedded in Araldite, and sectioned for LM
and EM autoradiography. Autoradiographs were prepared by
the dipping technique. Evaluation of the EM autoradiographs
was carried out using the circle method of Williams (for
details see Reisert and Pilgrim, 1979; Reisert et al., 1979).

Preferential accumulation of label in astrocytes as well
as in oligodendrocytes could be detected in LM and EM autoradiographs from 10 min to 2 hrs after injection of (^{3}H)
fucose. Similar observations were made in several hypothalamic areas as well as in thalamus, hippocampus, cerebellar
cortex, and hypoglossal nucleus. Table 1 gives the distribution of radioactivity in the supraoptic and arcuate nuclei

of the hypothalamus and the concentrations of radioactivity (grains/μm^2) in the three main tissue compartments, 30 min after application of (^{3}H)fucose. The smallest fraction of

Table 1. Data from EM autoradiographs of supraoptic and arcuate nuclei 30 min after L-(^{3}H)fucose.

Compartments	Radioactivity %[++]	Grains/μm^2
Neurons[+]	18.0	0.16 ± 0.02
Glia[+]	10.2	1.04 ± 0.13
Neuropil	58.4	0.01 ± 0.01

[+]Cell bodies

[++]Remaining structures
   (Cell nuclei, blood vessels, etc.)   13.4

radioactivity is found in the glia due to the fact that it is represented by few and small cell bodies only. However, it contains a high concentration of radioactivity which exceeds those of neuronal perikarya by a factor of 6.5. The reverse is true for the large compartment neuropil, i.e. the com- bined neuronal and glial processes. As to the types of glia involved, the data hold mostly for astroglia since it occupies by far the largest fraction of glial volume in grey matter.

   The time course of the incorporation pattern was followed after administration of (^{3}H)fucose (Reisert et al., 1977). Fig. 1 shows concentrations of radioactivity in glial cell bodies and neuropil relative to that of neurons. The data do not reveal significant differences in grain densities between astro- and oligodendroglia. The 30 min value in Fig. 1 does not quite conform to the glia/neuron ratio as it can be derived from Table 1. The reason is that, in the earlier set of experiments (Reisert et al., 1977), autoradio- graphs were used which were overexposed to some extent. This leads to an underestimation of grain densities in heavily labelled areas (Wagner et al., 1979). One observes a decrease of relative grain densities in glial cell bodies and an increase in the neuropil. Thus we have a shift of radioacti- vity from the cell bodies into the processes, and this seems to be more rapid on the expense of the glia than of the neurons. It is possible to conclude that the glia has a con- siderably higher rate of synthesis per unit volume as well as a higher turnover of glycoconjugates than neurons.

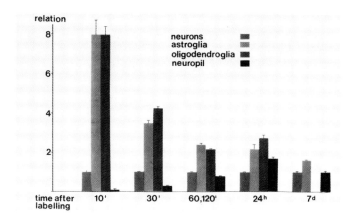

Fig. 1. Relative grain densities over cell bodies of neurons,
        glial cells and neuropil at various times after
        (^{3}H)fucose.

        Several experiments were run to confirm that the auto-
radiographic data truly reflect glycoconjugate metabolism.
The incorporation pattern of (^{3}H)fucose was compared with
that of another specific glycoconjugate precursor (^{3}H)N-
acetylmannosamine (Reisert and Pilgrim, 1979). The results

Table 2. Data from EM autoradiographs of the arcuate nucleus
         30 min after N-(^{3}H)acetyl-D-mannosamine.

Compartments	Radioactivity %[++]	Grains/μm^2
Neurons[+]	14.2	0.14 $\pm$ 0.01
Glia[+]	4.2	0.61 $\pm$ 0.13
Neuropil	71.8	0.08 $\pm$ 0.01

[+]Cell bodies
[++]Remaining structures
    (Cell nuclei, blood vessels, etc.)   9.8

closely resemble each other (cf. Tables 1 and 2), the grain
densities of glial cell bodies being 4.4. times higher than
those of neuronal perikarya. The fact that similar incorporation patterns were obtained with two different precursors
which are processed through different metabolic pathways
speaks for the above assumption. As the concentration of
radioactivity in the neuropil was relatively high after
(^{3}H)N-acetylmannosamine, an attempt was made in this set of
experiments to analyze the distribution of radioactivity
inside the neuropil. It could be shown that 46 % of the
radioactivity is held by glial, i.e. largely astroglial
processes.

Further evidence for the above interpretation of the
results is forthcoming when one compares these observations
with the data obtained after application of (^{3}H)leucine
(Reisert et al., 1979). As can be seen from Fig. 2, the
incorporation pattern is completely different. After (^{3}H)
leucine, the neuronal perikarya stand out against the

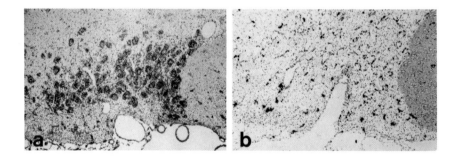

Fig. 2. LM autoradiographs of supraoptic nucleus 30 min
        after application of L-(^{3}H)leucine (a) and
        L-(^{3}H)fucose (b).
        Unstained, 180 x.

background, due to their well-known capacity for protein synthesis. After (^{3}H)fucose, one can hardly detect the neurons. Instead one observes small dense accumulations of silver grains which can be attributed to glial cell bodies. Table 3 provides the results of the quantitative evaluation.

Table 3. Data from EM autoradiographs of supraoptic and arcuate nuclei 30 min after L-(^{3}H)leucine.

Compartments	Radioactivity %[++]	Grains/μm^2
Neurons[+]	33.2	0.83 ± 0.22
Glia[+]	3.2	0.78 ± 0.12
Neuropil	48.6	0.12 ± 0.05

[+]Cell bodies

[++]Remaining structures
 (Cell nuclei, blood vessels, etc.)   15.0

In this case, the concentration of radioactivity in glial cell bodies relative to that of neurons is below 1.0.

Additional experiments support the notion that the radioactivity in the autoradiographs is due to macromolecular synthesis. It could be shown, for example, that non-enzymatic binding due to action of the aldehydes is non-existent with the radioactive monosaccharides (Ockenfels et al., in press). TCA-soluble radioactivity can be largely removed if the tissue is washed carefully after fixation (Reisert et al., in preparation).

Presently, the investigations are being extended to brain regions other than hypothalamus. The qualitative observations on the basis of LM autoradiographs cited above favour the assumption that the glia plays an important role in the glycoconjugate metabolism of several other brain regions as well. Preliminary quantitative results indicate, though, that there are regional variations. In the cerebellar cortex, for example, a lower glia/neuron ratio was found than in the two hypothalamic nuclei. This may turn out to be an interesting lead: depending on its location, the glia may express different states of activity.

It is known that most of the glycoconjugates in the
brain are localized in the intercellular space and/or on
the plasma membranes. Thus the active glycoconjugate metabolism in glial cells should be discussed with respect to
the size of plasma membranes. We have measured, by morpho-
metric techniques, the surface-to-volume ratio of the glial
and neuronal compartments in several parts of grey matter
(Pilgrim et al., in preparation). This value is, on the
average, twice as high for astroglia than for neurons. The
discrepancy becomes even more pronounced if one sets the
surface values in relation to the perikaryal volumes,
instead of the total volumes (cell bodies and processes).
Although these figures are not yet consistent enough, it
is probably justified to say that an astroglial perikaryon
has to take care of a several times larger surface than a
neuron. (One wonders whether the situation might not be
alike for the oligodendrocyte if one imagines that the
numerous loops of myelin be unrolled.) Since the capacity
for glycoconjugate synthesis is essentially confined to
the cell body, this spatial relationship could be one of
the reasons for the large glycoconjugate synthesizing
capacity of the glia.

Ockenfels H, Pilgrim Ch, Unsöld M (in press). In-vitro-
    Studien zur fixierungsbedingten Artefaktbildung in der
    elektronenmikroskopischen Autoradiographie. Acta histo-
    chem Suppl XXIV.
Pilgrim Ch, Wagner H-J (1975). Glycoprotein metabolism in
    the hypothalamus of rat: significance of glial cells.
    Histochemistry 45:289.
Reisert I, Pilgrim Ch (1979). Metabolism of glycoconjugates
    in hypothalamic neurons and glial cells: comparison of
    incorporation of (^{3}H)fucose and (^{3}H)N-acetylmannosamine
    by electron microscopic autoradiography. Cell Tissue
    Res 196:145.
Reisert I, Pilgrim Ch, Venedey Ch (1979). Incorporation of
    (^{3}H)leucine into hypothalamic nerve and glial cells. A
    comparison by EM autoradiography. Brain Research 172:521.
Reisert I, Wagner H-J, Pilgrim Ch (1977). Incorporation of
    ^{3}H-fucose into nerve and glial cells: assessment by
    electron microscopic autoradiography. J Comp Neurol
    176:453.
Wagner H-J, Reisert I, Möhler E, Pilgrim Ch (1979). Überex-
    position und Blockkontrastierung als Fehlerquellen der
    quantitativen Auswertung von elektronenmikroskopischen
    Autoradiogrammen. Acta histochem Suppl XX:107.

Eleventh International Congress of Anatomy:
Glial and Neuronal Cell Biology, pages 65—79
© **1981 Alan R. Liss, Inc., 150 Fifth Avenue, New York, NY 10011**

GLIAL FIBRILLARY ACIDIC (GFA) PROTEIN IMMUNOCYTOCHEMISTRY
IN DEVELOPMENT AND NEUROPATHOLOGY

Lawrence F. Eng and Stephen J. DeArmond

Department of Pathology, Veterans Administration
Med. Ctr., Palo Alto, CA. 94304, and Stanford
University School of Medicine, Stanford, CA 94305

An important mission of the Veterans Administration is
to care for patients with chronic neurological disorders
such as spinal cord injury, multiple sclerosis (MS), ischemic
vascular disease, aging, and dementia. A feature common to
all of these is extensive proliferation and hypertrophy of
astrocytes and their processes in cortical and subcortical
regions. The most prominent characteristic of astrocytic
gliosis is gliofibrillogenesis--the production of glial
filaments. Fundamental studies of the glial filament protein
are essential for our understanding of gliofibrillogenesis
and for any attempts to control astrocytic gliosis and to
promote spinal cord regeneration.

GFA PROTEIN: THE MAJOR PROTEIN CONSTITUENT OF GLIAL FILAMENTS

Since our initial isolation and characterization of the
glial fibrillary acidic (GFA) protein from MS plaques a
decade ago (Eng et al, 1970; Eng et al, 1971; for reviews see:
Eng & Bigbee, 1978, Eng, 1979, Eng, 1980 and Bignami et al,
1980), considerable evidence has accumulated which support
our view that the GFA protein is the major protein constituent
of glial filaments. Six lines of presumptive and direct
evidence which support our view are: (1) The GFA protein has
been isolated from nervous tissue known to be enriched with
fibrous astrocytes (i.e. MS plaques). (2) Antibody specific
to the GFA protein stains immunocytochemically only glial
fibril forming cells (astrocytes) at the light microscopic
level (Uyeda et al, 1972; Bignami et al, 1972; Ludwin et al,
1976). At the ultrastructural level, glial filaments are

prominently stained (Eng & Kosek, 1974; Schachner et al, 1977; Eng & Bigbee, 1978). (3) The 50,000 dalton protein from intermediate filaments isolated from normal bovine brain and spinal cord have very similar chemical and identical antigenic specificity to the GFA protein from MS plaques (DeVries et al, 1976; Eng et al, 1976). (4) In vitro biosynthesis of GFA protein employing mRNA from 16 day old mouse brain and immuno-precipitation with antiserum to bovine GFA protein yielded a single radiolabeled product with a MW of 50,000 daltons and a similar limited proteolytic peptide map as bovine and human GFA protein (Beguin et al, 1980). (5) Filaments reassembled in vitro from aqueous or 4M urea extracts of MS plaques have identical chemical and antigenic properties to purified GFA protein from MS plaques (Lucas et al, 1980) and stain positively at the ultrastructural level with the perox-idase-anti-peroxidase (PAP) method (Sternberger, 1979) employ-ing specific antibody to the GFA protein (Lucas et al, 1980). Filaments have also been reassembled from purified bovine GFA protein (Rueger et al, 1979). (6) Glial filaments isolated from human gliosed white matter have similar chemical and immunologic properties to GFA protein from MS plaques (Goldman et al, 1978).

RELATION OF GFA PROTEIN TO NEUROTUBULES AND NEUROFILAMENTS

Until recently considerable confusion existed concerning the chemical and immunological relationships between glial filament, neurofilament, and neurotubule proteins (Eng, 1980). Previously neurotubule protein had been reported to have similar chemical properties to glial filaments and GFA protein (Johnson & Sinex, 1974; Dahl, 1976a,b; Dahl & Bignami, 1976b; Chan et al, 1977). Neurotubules had also been reported to share common properties with neurofilaments (Wisniewski et al, 1968; Wisniewski et al, 1971; Gaskin & Shelanski, 1976; Iqbal et al, 1977). Antisera to a 54,000 MW protein isolated from chicken brain or human sciatic nerve have been reported to stain neurofilaments immunohistochemically (Dahl & Bignami, 1977). A recent study suggests that the major 54,000 MW protein of the chicken neurofilament preparation is tubulin, however minor proteins more antigenic than tubulin are also present since antiserum to this preparation reacts not only with the neurofilament proteins intensely, but also with a few other proteins including tubulin (Gambetti et al, 1980). Numerous other studies have suggested that neurofilament proteins share similar chemical and immunologic properties

with the GFA protein (Dahl & Bignami, 1976a; Yen et al, 1976;
Davison, 1975; Davison & Hong, 1977; Day, 1977; Goldman et al,
1978). For more details, see the recent reviews on neurofilaments (Schlaepfer, 1979; Shelanski & Liem, 1979; Norton
& Goldman, 1980). Presently it is generally agreed that the
GFA protein is chemically, morphologically, and antigentically
distinct from neurotubule and neurofilament proteins. Our
early reports (DeVries et al, 1976; Eng et al, 1976) were in
contention but have now been confirmed by many laboratories
(Bignami & Dahl, 1977; Liem et al, 1978; Schachner et al,
1978; Dahl & Bignami, 1979; Schlaepfer et al, 1979; Chiu
et al, 1980).

GFA PROTEIN IMMUNOCYTOCHEMISTRY AND MATURATION OF ASTROCYTES

An increased production of glial filaments characterizes
both the maturation of astrocytes and their response to
various pathological conditions in the central nervous
system. Various aspects of the synthesis and assembly of
glial filaments and their significance in relation to the
structure and function of the astrocyte, however, remain to
be established. A functional role for astrocytes and their
glial filaments has been suggested from two recent studies
which have employed GFA protein immunocytochemistry. Trimmer
et al (1979; 1980; 1980a) have recently described a tissue
culture system comprised of an enriched population of
immature and mature astrocytes from 5 to 7 day-old rat optic
nerves which they have used to study normal and drug-induced
astrocytic maturation in vitro with special emphasis on the
relationship between fibrillogenesis and glial development.
Maturation of selected astroblasts was followed in vitro by
phase contrast and differential-interference microscopy. At
different stages of maturation, these cells were fixed and
prepared for either immunocytochemical staining with anti-
GFA or for ultrastructural examination.

By phase contrast microscopy (Fig. la) two basic cell
types could be identified: (i) flat, polygonal, non-refractile
astroblasts and (ii) refractile, multipolar astrocytes. In
cultures which had been maintained for more than 20 days in
vitro, cells of intermediate morphology could also be identified. Immature, polygonal astroblasts in vitro did not
stain with anti-GFA (Fig. lb). At the ultrastructural level,
consistent with this lack of staining, astroblasts contained
few, if any, filaments and their general cytology resembled

that described in vivo. As maturation progressed in vitro, however, glial filaments gradually appeared in the perinuclear region of the astroblasts. Subsequently, distinct fascicles of glial filaments, which extended radially from the perinuclear region were distributed throughout the cytoplasm of the astroblasts. At slightly later stages, large cytoplasmic cavities, identifiable in living as well as anti-GFA stained cells, appeared between the radial bundles of filaments. As observed with the electron microscope, these cavities were consistently associated with numerous small vesicles, cisternae of smooth endoplasmic reticulum and microtubules. The consequence of this cytoplasmic cavitation was the erosion or retraction of cytoplasm between pre-established bundles of glial filaments. This maturational sequence ultimately gave rise to the formation of mature, multipolar astrocytes with filament-packed cellular processes (Fig. la, b). In addition to this sequence of process formation, astroglia in vitro demonstrated an ability to actively extend one or more processes for considerable distances from their cell bodies.

Dibutryl cyclic adenosine monophosphate (dbcAMP) has frequently been used to stimulate the formation of processes in immature astroblasts. In the present study, within a few hours after the addition of a lmM concentration of dbcAMP, astroblasts initiated the formation of processes. As was the case during normal maturation in vitro, extensive vacuolation occurred in the cytoplasm of dbcAMP-treated astroblasts. A regression of cytoplasm ensued as the vacuoles increased in size, leaving behind GFA-positive cellular processes. From these observations of normal and induced astrocytic differentiation in vitro, it appears that glial filaments participate in the formation of a cytoskeleton which may play an important role in defining the ultimate distribution of processes in the mature astrocyte. Whether or not this series of morphological changes reflects developmental processes in situ remains to be examined. In this regard, the possible role of neurites in regulating the maturation of astrocytes in situ must not be overlooked. Since these studies were conducted on isolated enriched cultures of astroglia, the absence of axon-glial interactions may conceivably account for any differences in astrocyte maturation in vivo as compared with in vitro. To this end, a study of gliogenesis in co-cultures should be undertaken to elucidate the influence of neuronal cell processes on astrocytic maturation.

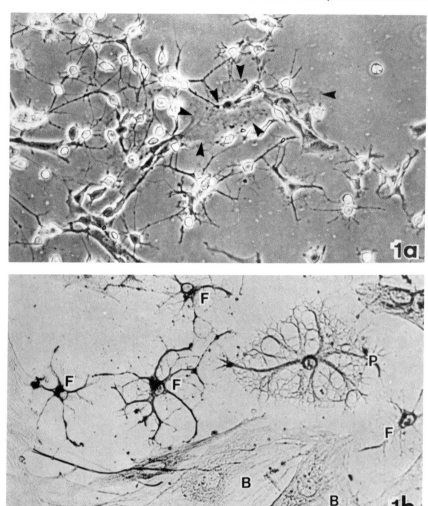

FIGURE la is a phase contrast micrograph of living astrocytes after 6 days in culture. The arrowheads indicate the
perimeter of a polygonal astroblast. Magnification - 100X.
FIGURE lb. Present in this light micrograph of a glial
culture stained with GFA antiserum after 98 days in vitro
are: four heavily stained fibrous astrocytes (f), one less
intensely stained protoplasmic astrocyte (p) and two
unstained, immature, polygonal astroblasts (b).
Magnification - 160X.

In a retrospective study, Levitt and Rakic (1980) stained rhesus monkey CNS from embryonic day 38 through the second postnatal month for the GFA protein. They reported that immunocytological localization of GFA in radial glial fibers at early stages of embryonic development indicated that glial cells were present concomitantly with neurons, raising the possibility that at least two distinct populations of cell precursors compose the proliferative zones. They further suggested that the presence of large numbers of radial glial cells in all brain regions during the peak of neuronal migration and a close structural relationship between elongated glial fibers and migrating neurons supported the concept that glial cells participate significantly in the guidance and compartmentalization of neuronal elements during development.

GFA PROTEIN IMMUNOCYTOCHEMISTRY AND RETROSPECTIVE PATHOLOGY

The PAP method of Sternberger has found wide application for research and clinical studies because of its extreme sensitivity and specificity. The high specificity of GFA protein antibody to glial filament forming cells has permitted us to apply immunocytochemical techniques to study fibrous gliosis in the CNS of aged, demented, and multiple sclerosis patients (Eng & Bigbee, 1978; Eng, et al, 1980) and to assist in the diagnosis of human brain tumors. The following is a brief summary of our findings.

The primary diseases of glial filament forming cells include neoplastic and nonneoplastic disorders. Since the first report on the use of peroxidase immunocytochemistry for GFA protein to examine human brain tumors (Deck et al, 1976), several others from this and other laboratories (Eng & Rubinstein, 1978; Deck et al, 1978; Kepes et al, 1979) have verified the original observations, established the technique as a crucial aid for the recognition of diagnostically difficult brain tumors, and have established the nature of a brain tumor of heretofore unknown nature. All of the studies to date have been reviewed recently (Eng & Bigbee, 1978; Eng, 1980; DeArmond et al, 1980) and the conclusions derived from them can be summarized as follows: (1) Neoplastic astrocytes stain positively for GFA protein with the intensity of staining roughly indirectly proportional to the degree of anaplasia of the neoplasm. Thus, well differentiated astrocytomas stain strongly while poorly differentiated astrocytomas of high grade malignancy stain only in their more differentiated regions. (2) Embryonal neuroepithelial neoplasms such as the medulloblastoma do not stain; however, regions of these neoplasms showing divergent differentiation to astrocytes are positive. (3) The technique clearly identifies the gliomatous regions of mixed tumors such as the gliosarcoma and ganglioglioma. (4) Although normal ependyma is negative, ependymomas can stain from strongly positive to negative. (5) The astroblastoma, a neoplasm of astrocytic lineage in which glial fibrils are typically absent, stains strongly for GFA protein. This observation indicates that glial filament formation is not a necessary consequence of GFA protein synthesis. (6) GFA immunocytochemistry has facilitated the diagnosis of gliomas which invaded the leptomeninges and induced the production of abundant connective tissue giving the false impression of a mesenchymal neoplasm. Similarly, we have been able to establish the glial nature of a distinctive supratentorial neoplasm previously interpreted as a fibrous xanthoma, now designated as pleomorphic xanthoastrocytoma. GFA protein has also been demonstrated in lipidized astrocytes in some hemangioblastomas of the CNS. (7) The GFA protein stain has been used to confirm the identity of gliomas metastasizing to extraneural sites and has been used to exclude non-glial neoplasms that may superficially resemble poorly differentiated forms of astrocytoma.

Only one disorder comes to mind that may represent a primary non-neoplastic disease of astrocytes, Alexander's disease. This rare disorder, regarded by Alexander (1949) as progressive fibrinoid degeneration of fibrillary astrocytes, is characterized by extensive fibrous gliosis with accumulation of Rosenthal fibers and diffuse demyelination in association with mental and neurological deterioration. Rosenthal fibers are rod-shaped homogeneous eosinophilic masses which can be 40 µ in length and 5 to 10 µ in diameter. In Alexander's disease, they preferentially accumulate in subpial and perivascular regions. By electron microscopy they are found within astrocytes and consist of homogeneous osmophilic granular masses which often appear to have glial filaments embedded in their outer surface and which tend to push other glial filaments aside. Two lines of evidence indicate that the basic defect in Alexander's disease occurs in astrocytes. First, the accumulation of Rosenthal fibers is generally believed to be a retrogressive change since they are commonly found in regions of long standing fibrous

gliosis, such as in slowly-growing astrocytomas, and in
long-standing reactive gliosis as is associated with multiple
sclerosis plaques or CNS infarcts. Second, the deposition
of Rosenthal fibers is usually more widespread than the demyelination of white matter. Histochemical evidence indicates
that Rosenthal fibers contain an insoluble digestion resistant
protein (Herndon et al, 1970). We are currently attempting
to isolate the protein from a case of Alexander's disease
(Ramsay, Norman and Eng, 1979). Immunocytochemistry of
Rosenthal fibers from cases of Alexander's disease, multiple
sclerosis and an astrocytoma indicate that the bulk of their
mass does not contain GFA protein, myelin basic protein or
tubulin. However, the periphery of the mass stains positively for GFA protein presumably because of the glial filaments
present at the surface (Eng and Bigbee, 1978; Eng, Norman,
Bigbee and Rubinstein, unpublished data). At this time the
identity of the protein and etiology of the disease remain
unknown.

The study of secondary or reactive gliosis by GFA
protein immunocytochemistry has both clarified and confirmed
the concepts derived from classical neurohistological techniques for glial fibrils such as the Holzer stain. However,
certain critical differences exist between the two techniques.
Immunocytochemistry is highly specific for GFA protein and
consequently stains only glial filament forming cells. In
contrast, the Holzer stain, while highly specific for glial
fibrils (presumably bundles of glial filaments), also stains
blood vessels and cell nuclei; it does not stain the non-
fibrillated component of the astrocyte cytoplasm. GFA
immunocytochemistry strongly stains the astrocyte perikaryon
and only weakly stains glial fibrils and processes packed
with glial fibrils. We believe that the GFA protein staining
pattern reflects the presence of unpolymerized GFA, which is
presumably diffusely cytoplasmic, while GFA polymerized into
filaments has fewer exposed antigenically reactive sites(Fig.2)
(DeArmond et al, 1980). Furthermore the number of GFA-
containing normal astrocytes which stain depends on the method
of tissue processing which may denature the antigen. A larger
number of astrocytes stain in a frozen section than in a comparable section which has been fixed and embedded routinely.

GFA immunocytochemistry has demonstrated GFA protein
synthesis by both protoplasmic and fibrous astrocytes in
response to brain injury. An example of the reactivity of
protoplasmic astrocytes is their response to a stab wound

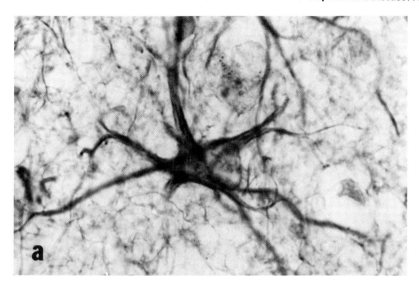

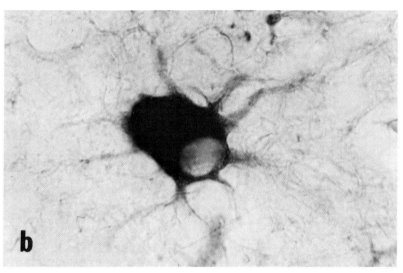

FIGURE 2. Reactive astrocytes in the human cerebral cortex.
a. Holzer stain reveals the network of glial fibers coursing
through the cytoplasm and extending far distally into astrocytic processes. X1000. b. Immunoperoxidase technique for
GFA protein stains the cell cytoplasm and proximal portions of
astrocytic processes. X1000. (Sections were prepared by Mr.
Robert McGowan in Dr. Lucien Rubinstein's laboratory)

in the cerebral cortex. Although normal ependyma does not stain for GFA protein, the technique has demonstrated that reactive ependyma, which contains 80 to 90 Å filaments resembling glial filaments, becomes strongly GFA positive (Deck et al, 1978).

The occurrence of GFA protein in peripheral nerve has also been investigated in normal and disease states. It is well known that true CNS tissue containing oligodendrocytes, central myelin and astrocytes protrude into nerve roots at the CNS-PNS transition region, especially in lumbar nerve roots and most dramatically in the eighth cranial nerve. The CNS border is sharply delineated in this region by the glial limiting membrane composed of specialized astrocytic processes covered by a basement membrane. Only two structures of CNS origin are found distal to the membrane in the normal state: axons derived from anterior horn cells and the sympathetic column and delicate astrocytic processes. The latter are termed the glial fringe and normally do not protrude more than a fraction of a millimeter beyond the membrane. The bundles of glial processes forming the fringe are encased in a basement membrane which is continuous with that overlying the limiting membrane. The fringe is not present in infants and appears to develop in response to axonal injury and loss. Proliferation and extension of the glial fringe to as far as 2 cm from the CNS-PNS junction was once believed to be pathognomonic of Werdnig-Hoffmann disease, a uniformly fatal spinal-muscular atrophy of infancy with extensive loss of large motorneurons (Chou and Nonaka, 1978; Ghatak, 1978). GFA immunocytochemistry (Chou et al, 1979) demonstrated that these bundles are strongly GFA positive and are present in the posterior as well as anterior roots. Although the glial fringe has not been found to proliferate in amyotrophic lateral sclerosis or the Guillain-Barre syndrome (DeArmond et al, 1980a), abnormal extension of glial bundles into pheripheral nerves has been reported to occur in poliomyelitis (Iwata & Hirano, 1978) and following sectioning of spinal nerve roots in the pig (Meier & Sollmann, 1978). The former authors do not describe the full extent of the abnormal astrocytic fringe protrusion into the peripheral nerve; the latter report astrocytic processes extended 2 cm from the CNS-PNS junction. All GFA staining in peripheral nerve we have seen to date has been localized to nerve roots and was attributable to extrusion of astrocytic processes. We have never observed staining of Schwann cells.

ACKNOWLEDGEMENTS: Our studies reported here were supported in part by the VA and NIH grant (NS-11632). We thank Ms. Donna Buckley for technical assistance; Drs. Trimmer, Reier, Oh, Levitt, and Rakic for their reports which are in press; and Drs. Chou and H.H. Goebel for tissues and unpublished data.

REFERENCES

Beguin P, Shooter EM, Eng LF (1980). Cell-free synthesis of glial fibrillary acidic protein. Neurochem Res 5:513-521.

Bignami A, Dahl D (1977). Specificity of the glial fibrillary acidic protein for astroglia. J Histochem Cytochem 25:466-469.

Bignami A, Dahl D, Rueger DC (1980). Glial fibrillary acidic GFA Protein in normal neural cells and in pathological conditions. In Federoff S, Hertz L (eds): "Advances in Cellular Neurobiology Vol 1," New York: Academic Press, pp 285-310.

Bignami A, Eng LF, Dahl D, Uyeda CT (1972). Localization of the glial fibrillary acidic protein in astrocytes by immuno-fluorescence. Brain Res 43:429-435.

Chan PH, Huston JS, Moo-penn WF, Dahl D, Bignami A (1977). Biochemical studies related to CNS regeneration: Isolation and partial characterization of urea-soluble gliofibrillary acidic protein from bovine brain. In: "Proceedings of the Second Annual Maine Biomedical Science Symposium, V II," University of Maine Press, pp 496-524.

Chiu F-C, Korey B, Norton WT (1980). Intermediate filaments from bovine rat and human CNS: Mapping analysis of the major protein. J Neurochem 34(5):1149-1159.

Chou SM, Miike T, Eng LF (1979). Studies of glial bundles in Werdnig-Hoffman Disease (WHD) by the immunoperoxidase method. J Neuropath Exp Neurol 38:307.

Chou SM, Nonaka I (1978). Werdnig-Hoffmann Disease: proposal of a pathogenetic mechanism. Acta Neuropath 41:45-54.

Dahl D (1976a). Glial fibrillary acidic protein from bovine and rat brain. Degradation in tissues and homogenates. Biochim Biophys Acta 420:142-154.

Dahl D (1976b). Isolation and initial characterization of glial fibrillary acidic protein from chicken, turtle, frog, and fish central nervous system. Biochim Biophys Acta 446:41-50.

Dahl D, Bignami A (1976a). Isolation from peripheral nerve of a protein similar to the glial fibrillary acidic protein. FEBS Letters 66:281-284.

Dahl D, Bignami A (1976b). Immunogenic properties of the glial fibrillary acidic protein. Brain Res 116:150-157.

Dahl D, Bignami A (1977). Preparation of antisera to neurofilament protein from chicken brain and human sciatic nerve. J Comp Neur 176:645-657.

Dahl D, Bignami A (1979). Astroglial and axonal proteins in isolated brain filaments. Biochim Biophys Acta 578:305-316.

Davison PF (1975). Neuronal fibrillar proteins and axoplasmic transport. Brain Res 100:73-80.

Davison PF, Hong B-S (1977). Structural homologies in mammalian neurofilament proteins. Brain Res 134:287-295.

Day WA (1977). Solubilization of neurofilaments from central nervous system myelinated nerve. J Ultrastruct Res 60: 362-372.

DeArmond SJ, Deibler GE, Bacon M, Kies MW, Eng LF (1980a). A neurochemical and immunocytochemical study of P-2 protein in human and bovine nervous systems. J Histochem Cytochem. In press.

DeArmond SJ, Eng LF, Rubinstein LJ (1980). The application of glial fibrillary acidic (GFA) protein immunohistochemistry in neurooncology: a progress report. Path Res Pract 168: 374-394.

Deck JH, Eng LF, Bigbee J (1976). A preliminary study of glioma morphology using the peroxidase-anti-peroxidase method for the GFA protein. J Neuropath Exp Neurol 35:362.

Deck JHN, Eng LF, Bigbee J, Woodcock SM (1978). The role of glial fibrillary acidic protein in the diagnosis of central nervous system tumours. Acta Neuropathol Berl 42:183-190.

DeVries GH, Eng LF, Lewis DH, Hadfield MG (1976). The protein composition of bovine myelin-free axons. Biochim Biophys Acta 439:133-145.

Eng LF (1979). Reply to the comments of Bignami and Dahl. J Histochem Cytochem 27:694-696.

Eng LF (1980). The glial fibrillary acidic (GFA) protein. In Bradshaw RA, Schneider DM (eds): "Proteins of the Nervous System, 2nd ed," New York: Raven Press, pp 85-117.

Eng LF, Bigbee JW (1978). Immunohistochemistry of nervous system-specific antigens. In Agranoff BW, Aprison MH (eds): "Advances in Neurochemistry," Vol 3, New York: Plenum Press, pp 43-98.

Eng LF, DeVries GH, Lewis DL, Bigbee JW (1976). Specific antibody to the major 47,000 MW protein fraction of bovine myelin-free axons. Fed Proc 35:1766.

Eng LF, Forno LS, Bigbee JW, Forno KI (1980). Immunocytochemical localization of glial fibrillary acidic protein and tubulin in Alzheimer's disease brain biopsy tissue. In

Amaducci L, Davison AN, Antuono P (eds): "Aging of the Brain and Dementia", New York: Raven Press, pp 49-54.

Eng LF, Gerstl B, Vanderhaeghen JJ (1970). A study of proteins in old multiple sclerosis plaques. Trans Am Soc Neurochem 1:42.

Eng LF, Kosek JC (1974). Light and electron microscopic localization of the glial fibrillary acidic protein and S-100 protein by immunoenzymatic techniques. Trans Am Soc Neurochem 5:160.

Eng LF, Rubinstein LJ (1978). Contribution of immunohistochemistry to diagnostic problems of human cerebral tumors. J Histochem Cytochem 26:513-522.

Eng LF, Vanderhaeghen JJ, Bignami A, Gerstl B (1971). An acidic protein isolated from fibrous astrocytes. Brain Res 28:351-354.

Gambetti P, Velasco ME, Dahl D, Bignami A, Roessmann U, and Sindely SD (1980). Alzheimer neurofibrillary tangles: An immunohistochemical study. In Amaducci L, Davison AN, Antuono P (eds): "Aging of the Brain and Dementia", New York: Raven Press, pp 55-63.

Gaskin F, Shelanski ML (1976). Microtubules and intermediate filaments. Essays in Biochemistry 12:115-146.

Ghatak NR (1978). Spinal roots in Werdnig-Hoffmann disease. Acta Neuropath 41:1-7.

Goldman JE, Schaumburg HH, Norton WT (1978). Isolation and characterization of glial filaments and neurofilaments from human brain. Similarity of the major protein components. J Cell Biol 78:426-444.

Herndon RM, Rubinstein LJ, Freeman JM, Mathieson G (1970). Light and electron microscopic observations on Rosenthal fibers in Alexander's disease and in multiple sclerosis. J Neuropath Exp Neurol 29:524-551.

Iqbal K, Grundke-Iqbal I, Wisniewski HM, Terry RD (1977). On neurofilament and neurotubule proteins from human autopsy tissue. J Neurochem 29:417-424.

Iwata M, Hirano A (1978). "Glial Bundles" in the spinal cord late after paralytic anterior poliomyelitis. Ann Neurol 4: 562-563.

Johnson L, Sinex FM (1974). On the relationship of brain filaments to microtubules. J Neurochem 22:321-326.

Kepes JJ, Rubinstein LJ, Eng LF (1979). Pleomorphic xanthoastrocytoma. A distinctive meningocerebral glioma of young subjects with relatively favorable prognosis. A study of 12 cases. Cancer 44:1839-1852.

Levitt P, Rakic P (1980). Immunoperoxidase localization of glial fibrillary acidic protein in radial glial cells and astrocytes of the developing rhesus monkey brain. J Comp Neur. In press.

Liem RKH, Yen SH, Salomon GD, Shelanski ML (1978). Intermediate filaments in nervous tissue. J Cell Biol 79:637-645.

Lucas CV, Bensch KG, Eng LF (1980). In vitro polymerization of the glial fibrillary acidic (GFA) protein extracted from multiple sclerosis (MS) brain. Neurochem Res 5:247-255.

Lucas CV, Reaven EP, Bensch KG, Eng LF (1980). Immunoperoxidase staining of glial fibrillary acidic (GFA) protein polymerized in vitro: an ultramicroscopic study. Neurochem Res. In press.

Ludwin SK, Kosek JC, Eng LF (1976). The topographical distribution of S-100 and GFA proteins in the adult rat brain: An immunohistochemical study using horseradish peroxidase-labeled antibodies. J Comp Neurol 165:197-208.

Meier C, Sollmann H (1978). Glial outgrowth and central-type myelination of regenerating axons in spinal nerve roots following transection and suture: light and electron microscopic study in the pig. Neuropath Appl Neurobiol 4:21-35.

Norton WT, Goldman JE (1980). Neurofilaments. In Bradshaw RA, Schneider DW (eds): "Proteins of the Nervous System, 2nd ed," New York: Raven Press.

Ramsay P, Norman M, Eng LF (1979). Chemical study of an Alexander's brain. Trans Am Soc Neurochem 10:110.

Rueger DC, Huston JS, Dahl D, Bignami A (1979). Formation of 100 Å filaments from purified glial fibrillary acidic protein in vitro. J Mol Biol 135:53-68.

Schachner M, Hedley-Whyte ET, Hsu DW, Schoonmaker G, Bignami A (1977). Ultrastructural localization of glial fibrillary acidic protein in mouse cerebellum by immunoperoxidase labeling. J Cell Biol 75:67-73.

Schachner M, Smith C, Schoonmaker G (1978). Immunological distinction between neurofilament and glial fibrillary acidic protein by mouse antisera and their immunohistological characterization. Dev Neurosci 1:1-14.

Schlaepfer WW (1979). Nature of mammalian neurofilaments and their breakdown by calcium. In Zimmerman HM (ed): "Progress in Neuropathology, Vol 4," New York: Raven Press, pp 101-123.

Schlaepfer WW, Freeman LA, Eng LF (1979). Studies of human and bovine spinal nerve roots and the evagination of CNS tissues into the nerve root entry zone. Brain Res 177:219-229.

Shelanski ML, Liem RKH (1979). Neurofilaments. J Neurochem 33:5-13.

Sternberger LA (1979). "Immunocytochemistry" Second Edition. New York: John Wiley & Sons, Inc.

Trimmer PA, Reier PJ, Oh TH (1979). Tissue culture of normal astrocytes from rat optic nerve. Soc Neurosci 5:780. Abst.

Trimmer PA, Reier PJ, Oh TH (1980). Morphological studies of normal and induced astrocytic differentiation in vitro. Soc Neurosci 6. In press.

Trimmer PA, Reier PJ, Oh TH, Eng LF (1980a). Maturation of mammalian astrocytes. In vitro: Ultrastructural and immuno-cytochemical study. In preparation.

Uyeda CT, Eng LF, Bignami A (1972). Immunological study of the glial fibrillary acidic protein. Brain Res 37:81-89.

Wisniewski H, Shelanski ML, Terry RD (1968). Effects of mito-tic spindle inhibitors on neurotubules and neurofilaments in anterior horn cells. J Cell Biol 38:224-229.

Wisniewski H, Terry RC, Hirano A (1971). Neurofibrillary pathology. J Neuropath Exp Neurol 29:173-181.

Yen SH, Dahl D, Schachner M, Shelanski ML (1976). Biochemistry of the filaments of brain. Proc Nat Acad Sci USA 73:529-533.

STRUCTURE AND FUNCTION
OF OLIGODENDROCYTES

Eleventh International Congress of Anatomy:
Glial and Neuronal Cell Biology, pages 83—92
© **1981 Alan R. Liss, Inc., 150 Fifth Avenue, New York, NY 10011**

POSTNATAL DEVELOPMENT OF OLIGODENDROCYTES

J.A. PATERSON

DEPARTMENT OF ANATOMY
UNIVERSITY OF MANITOBA
WINNIPEG, MANITOBA, CANADA

In developing nervous tissue, the time when the most rapid production of oligodendrocytes occurs differs with species and with different regions of the central nervous system; this time of abundant oligodendrocyte production seems to parallel the time of rapid myelination in that region (Phillips, '73; Privat '75; Skoff et al., '76a,b; Sturrock, '76; Varon and Somjen, '79). The rodent corpus callosum, a cerebral commissure myelinated during the first month of life, is one of the regions rich in oligodendrocytes produced postnatally. In the cerebrum of rodents, the postnatal genesis of astrocytes and oligodendrocytes begins at subventricular sites where mitotically-active cells are clustered; such a site is the subependymal layer of the anterior horn of the lateral ventricle. The production of neuroglial precursors and their migration from subependymal layer to adjacent regions occurs at a rapid rate during the first few weeks of life, and continues into adulthood (Smart, '61; Altman,'66; Lewis, '68). Radioautographic evidence indicates a subependymal origin for the immature glial precursor cells observed in the corpus callosum of young rats (Privat and Leblond, '72; Paterson et al., '73) and also indicates that the oligodendrocyte in its passage from dividing precursor to mature form, progresses gradually through a sequence of morphological changes (Paterson et al., '73; Imamoto et al., '78).

MORPHOLOGY OF THE OLIGODENDROCYTE LINE

As recognized by Kruger and Maxwell ('66) and Mori and
Leblond ('70), the oligodendrocyte class includes cells varying from large and pale to small and dense, yet all sharing
the common features of one family. These cells can be accurately identified by their appearance in semithin plastic
sections stained with toluidine blue, as well as by their
ultrastructure (Mori and Leblond, '70; Ling et al., '73).
The three main subclasses of oligodendrocyte are illustrated
in semithin section (fig. 1).

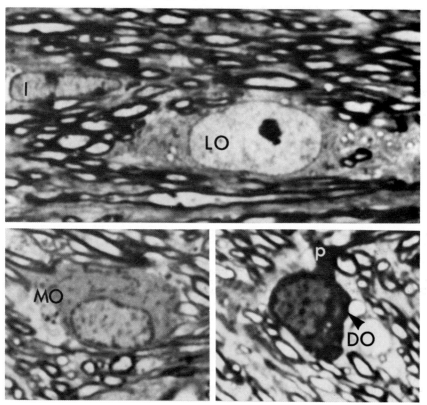

Fig. 1. Oligodendrocytes in corpus callosum of rats after
   aldehyde fixation. An immature-looking cell is at I.
   Plastic section, toluidine blue stain. x 3000
   (from Ling et al., '73. Reproduced with permission of
   Wistar Institute Press).

In semithin section, the *light oligodendrocyte* (LO) has a pale, oval nucleus with a prominent nucleolus and dispersed chromatin. The perikaryon is abundant and lightly basophilic. The *dark oligodendrocyte* (DO) has a small, often indented nucleus containing patches of condensed chromatin; its nucleoplasm and especially its cytoplasm are basophilic. The cytoplasm, reduced in volume, may collect asymmetrically around the nucleus, with few visible extensions into processes (p). The *medium oligodendrocyte* (MO) has a nucleus and perikaryon intermediate in size and moderate in basophilia. In young rats, there are many cells intermediate in form between the light and the dark cells, so that a continuous series of sizes and densities is found.

Electron microscopy confirms the finding of a spectrum of oligodendrocytes showing a progressive reduction in the size, and an increase in electron density, of nucleus and cytoplasm. The oligodendrocytes as a class have abundant cytoplasmic organelles: Golgi bodies, vesicles, ribosomes, narrow cisternae of rough endoplasmic reticulum, mitochondria and microtubules; and they all lack the glycogen and filaments characteristic of astrocytes. The light oligodendrocyte (fig. 2) is rich in polysomes, free and bound. The cisternae of rough endoplasmic reticulum occur both singly and aligned in stacks of three or four. This stacking of cisternae becomes increasingly evident in the medium and dark cells. The characteristic cytoplasmic processes, containing microtubules, are more plentiful in the light than in the medium and dark cells (fig. 3). The light cell has chromatin in fine loose patches throughout the pale nucleoplasm; the medium cell and dark cell show increased clumping of chromatin. The light cell has a cytoplasmic matrix only slightly more electron dense than that of an astrocyte or neuron, whereas the medium and dark cells show a greater cytoplasmic density (fig. 4); the constituent that imparts this density is not known. The organelles in the dark cells appear "crowded" into a much more compact arrangement than the scattered profusion they show in the light and medium oligodendrocytes; this compactness is a constant feature of dark cells (Leblond, personal communication). Membraneous and other inclusion bodies are also typical of dark cells (Vaughan and Peters, '74).

In rats three weeks of age, the corpus callosum contains among its neuroglia the three types of oligodendrocytes, as well as the *immature cells* common in young rats (Ling et al.,

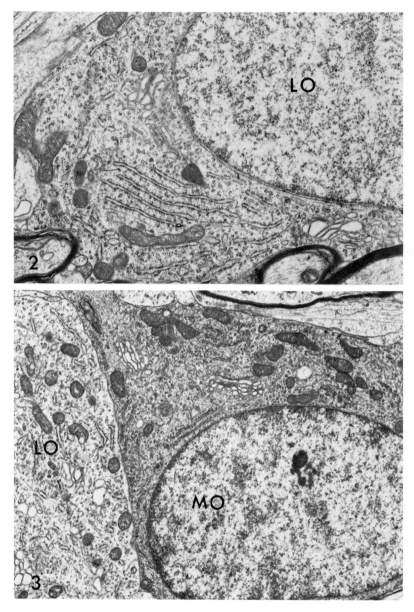

Oligodendrocytes in 7 wk old rat. Fig. 2. Light oligodendrocyte (LO) x 16,000. Fig. 3. The cell at right is intermediate in features between a medium and dark oligodendrocyte. Compare with dark cell in fig. 4. x 11,200.

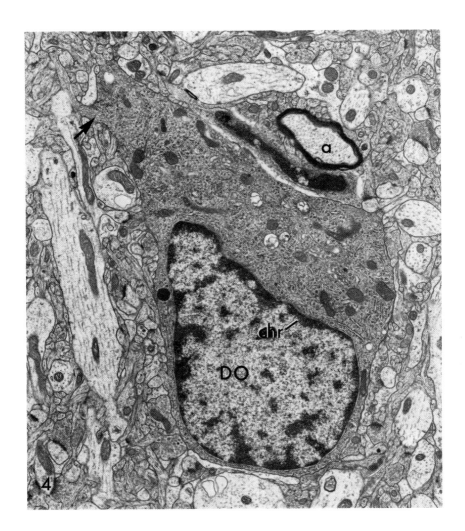

Fig. 4. Dark oligodendrocyte in cerebral cortex of 7-wk old
rat. Note chromatin clumping (chr) in eccentrically
located nucleus. Ribosomes and other organelles appear in
the compact perikaryon, whose relatively-regular margin is
discernible. Fine processes contain microtubules (arrow).
A small part of another cell nucleus is adjacent and a
myelinated axon is nearby (a). x 11,000.

'73; Sturrock, '76; Imamoto et al., '78). The immature cells constitute about one fifth of glia in corpus callosum at three weeks of age, but later their percentage decreases to about 2% by three months. The term "immature cell" in light microscopic descriptions denotes a member of a group of morphologically undifferentiated or incompletely differentiated cells. Some such cells have a small elongated nucleus surrounded by a thin rim of cytoplasm, while others have irregular-shaped or larger rounded nuclei with visible nucleolus and chromatin patchiness. (see I in figure 1). The heterogenity of this immature class is confirmed by ultrastructural study. Some of these cells have an abundance of ribosomes in their scanty, slightly dense cytoplasm, but few other organelles. Others of the immature cells appear to have some features of astrocytes, while others appear to have some oligodendrocyte characteristics (Privat and Leblond, '72; Skoff et al., '76a; Imamoto et al., '78). With the light microscope, however, the distinction between these types of immature cells is difficult.

The subependymal layer contains many cells with the ultrastructural features of undifferentiated cells (Blakemore, '69; Privat and Leblond, '72; Sturrock and Smart, '80). In young rats, part of this complex, mitotically-active cell group extends laterally between corpus callosum and caudate nucleus, and apparently undifferentiated and partly differentiated cells appear in this extension, as well as in the corpus callosum.

RADIOAUTOGRAPHIC EVIDENCE FOR THE SUBEPENDYMAL ORIGIN AND SEQUENTIAL DEVELOPMENT OF OLIGODENDROCYTES IN CORPUS CALLOSUM

In one-month old rats given an intraventricular injection of ^{3}H-thymidine, many of the dividing subependymal cells became radioactively-labeled at the time of the injection; and labeled cells were detected, at later time intervals after the injection, in increasing numbers outside of the subependymal layer (Lewis, '68; Paterson et al., '73). These cells that had migrated were identified at early and later times after injection. From this work, the subependymal origin of the immature-looking cells found in corpus callosum was evident, and their role as glial precursors was indicated. Many of these cells became oligodendrocytes, and a few became astrocytes; the production of most astrocytes in corpus callosum probably occurs at an earlier age than this (Sturrock, '76).

The development of oligodendrocytes in corpus callosum of three week old rats given intraperitoneal injections of ^{3}H-thymidine was analysed by light microscopic radioautography (Imamoto et al., '78). In rats killed *two hours* after injection, the radioactively-labeled cells were those that had been preparing to divide at the time of the injection. In the subependymal layer, 16% of cells were labeled. In the corpus callosum, only the immature cells had many labeled members, that is, members that were dividing (10%). This labeled immature group contained both apparently undifferentiated and partly differentiated cells. Among the oligodendrocytes, the light, medium and dark cells showed essentially no labeling. That none of the oligodendrocytes were dividing was in agreement with the ultrastructural study of optic nerve by Skoff et al. ('76a), who observed that among the oligodendrocytes only their immature partly differentiated precursors were dividing.

Imamoto and co-workers then examined the progeny of the immature cells that were labeled, in rats that were killed at longer time intervals after ^{3}H-thymidine injection. The cells showing label at the later times were identified, and the per cent cells labeled of each type was calculated and plotted against time (fig. 5).

The time plot shows that the per cent of labeled immature cells rises rapidly and then drops. This cell group increases both by its own divisions and by the influx of cells (many of which would be labeled) from the subependymal region (Privat and Leblond, '72). The subsequent drop in labeling per cent suggests that many of the immature cells, including labeled ones, are leaving this group, by transforming into cells of another type. Meanwhile, labeled cells appear in the nonproliferating light oligodendrocyte group, first at two days post injection, and increasingly until seven days. Comparing the pattern of labeling in these two cell groups suggests that many of the immature cells are transforming into light oligodendrocytes. In the medium oligodendrocyte group, labeled cells appear and the labeling percentage reaches a peak a few days *later* than the peak for light cells. Labeled dark oligodendrocytes are the last to appear, in gradually greater numbers. This sequential pattern of labeling peaks indicates that there is a successive transformation of cells, with light oligodendrocytes transforming into medium cells, and medium cells becoming dark oligodendrocytes, the final stage. Thus the

three classes of oligodendrocyte represent stages in a
developmental sequence.

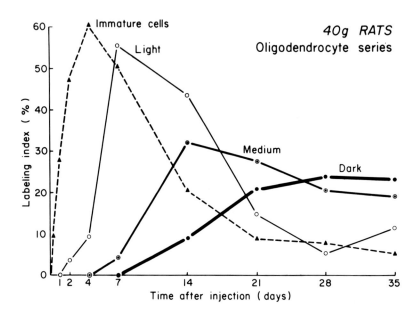

Fig. 5. (from Imamoto, Paterson and Leblond, '78. Reproduced by permission of Wistar Institute Press).

The proportions of the types of oligodendrocytes present
in corpus callosum are observed to differ between young and
adult rat, an observation compatible with the developmental
scheme. Light oligodendrocytes, present during the second
postnatal week (Sturrock, '76) are abundant during the third
week, when medium cells are also common and dark cells are
few. With increasing age, the proportion of light and medium
cells decreases, while that of dark oligodendrocytes increases until about 3.5 months of age, after which their
number is maintained, in corpus callosum (Ling and Leblond,
'73) and in cortex (Vaughan and Peters, '74). Still in
adulthood, a few members of the oligodendrocyte group may be
observed at the light stage, while most others are at later
stages of the developmental progression. Also, a very small
percentage of immature cells are observed in adult corpus
callosum (Ling and Leblond, '73; Sturrock, '76).

The ultrastructural and radioautographic studies described above may be summarized in the following proposal. Proliferative immature cells leave the subependymal layer, and some enter the corpus callosum, as glial precursors. These glial precursors may be in the form of small cells with an undifferentiated appearance--glioblasts--which may serve as intermediaries between subependymal cells and later stages. In a sequence that is not yet clear, partly differentiated oligodendrocyte precursors (oligodendroblasts) are formed among the proliferative immature cells. An oligodendroblast, following its last division, becomes the large, light oligodendrocyte. After a few days in this form, this cell develops into a medium oligodendrocyte, a stage that occupies about two weeks. Gradually the medium cell assumes the form of the smaller, dark oligodendrocyte; this form is the mature and long lasting stage in the development of oligodendrocytes (Imamoto et al., '78).

REFERENCES

Altman J (1966). Proliferation and migration of undifferentiated precursor cells in the rat during postnatal gliogenesis. Exp Neurol 16:263.

Blakemore WF (1969). The ultrastructure of the subependymal plate in the rat. J Anat 104:423.

Imamoto K, Paterson J, Leblond CP (1978). Radioautographic investigation of gliogenesis in the corpus callosum of young rats. I. Sequential changes in oligodendrocytes. J Comp Neur 180:115.

Kruger L, Maxwell DS (1966). Electron microscopy of oligodendrocytes in normal rat cerebrum. Amer J Anat 118:411.

Lewis PD (1968). The fate of the subependymal cell in the adult rat brain, with a note on the origin of microglia. Brain 91:721.

Ling EA, Leblond CP (1973). Investigation of glial cells in semithin sections. II. Variation with age in the numbers of the various glial cell types in rat cortex and corpus callosum. J Comp Neur 149:73.

Ling EA, Paterson JA, Privat A, Mori S, Leblond CP (1973). Investigation of glial cells in semithin sections. I. Identification of glial cells in the brain of young rats. J Comp Neur 149:43.

Mori S, Leblond CP (1970). Electron microscopic identification of three classes of oligodendrocytes and a preliminary study of their proliferative activity in the corpus callosum of young rats. J Comp Neur 139:1.

Paterson JA, Privat A, Ling EA, Leblond CP (1973). Investigation of glial cells in semithin sections. III. Transformation of subependymal cells into glial cells, as shown by radioautography after ^{3}H-thymidine injection into the lateral ventricle of the brain of young rats. J Comp Neur 149:83.

Phillips DE (1973). An electron microscopic study of macroglia and microglia in the lateral funiculus of the developing spinal cord in the fetal monkey. Z Zellforsch 140:145.

Privat A (1975). Postnatal gliogenesis in the mammalian brain. Int Rev Cytol 40:281.

Privat A, Leblond CP (1972). The subependymal layer and neighbouring region in the brain of the young rat. J Comp Neur 146:277.

Skoff RP, Price DL, Stocks A (1976a). Electron microscopic autoradiographic studies of gliogenesis in rat optic nerve. I. Cell proliferation. J Comp Neur 169:291.

Skoff RP, Price DL, Stocks A (1976b). Electron microscopic autoradiographic studies of gliogenesis in rat optic nerve. II. Time of origin. J Comp Neur 169:313.

Smart I (1961). The subependymal layer of the mouse brain and its cell production as shown by radioautography after ^{3}H-thymidine injection. J Comp Neur 116:325.

Sturrock RR (1976). Light microscopic identification of immature glial cells in semithin sections of the developing mouse corpus callosum. J Anat 122:521.

Sturrock RR, Smart IHM (1980). A morphological study of the mouse subependymal layer from embryonic life to old age. J Anat 130:391.

Varon SS, Somjen GG (1979). "Neuron-glia interactions." Neurosciences Res Prog Bull 17. Cambridge: MIT Press.

Vaughan DW, Peters A (1974). Neuroglial cells in the cerebral cortex of rats from young adulthood to old age: an electron microscopic study. J Neurocytol 3:405.

Eleventh International Congress of Anatomy:
Glial and Neuronal Cell Biology, pages 93–103
© 1981 Alan R. Liss, Inc., 150 Fifth Avenue, New York, NY 10011

PROLIFERATION OF OLIGODENDROGLIAL CELLS IN NORMAL ANIMALS
AND IN A MYELIN DEFICIENT MUTANT-JIMPY

ROBERT P. SKOFF

DEPARTMENT OF ANATOMY, WAYNE STATE UNIVERSITY
SCHOOL OF MEDICINE, 540 E. CANFIELD
DETROIT, MI 48201

PROLIFERATION OF OLIGODENDROGLIAL CELLS IN NORMAL DEVELOPMENT

The lineage of neuroglial cells in the central nervous
system (CNS) has been investigated since 1889, when His began
his original study. Different schemes have been proposed
from these studies (e.g., Vaughn, '69; Phillips, '73;
Sturrock, '74) and many questions remain unanswered. For
example, do astrocytes and oligodendrocytes arise from a
multipotential stem cell or are there separate cell lines for
each? There are many reasons why the progress in analyzing
gliogenesis has been slow but one which we believe very
important centers around the methods used to study neuroglia.
Since glial cells are considerably smaller than neurons, it
is difficult to accurately classify the different cell types
with the light microscope. It is even more difficult to
document transitional stages in their development.
Furthermore, cells about to undergo cell division cannot be
identified by microscopy alone but require a chemical
indicator. Many of the problems inherent in the study of
gliogenesis can be overcome by combining electron microscopy
with ^{3}H-thymidine autoradiographic techniques. The
resolution of electron microscopy allows for an accurate
description of neuroglia while radioactive thymidine (a
precursor for DNA) may be used to directly mark cells during
their proliferative periods. Cells about to enter mitosis
can be identified in autoradiograms from animals sacrificed
shortly after an injection of ^{3}H-thymidine. The time of
origin for neuroglia can be determined using autoradiographic
techniques similar to those used in dating the origin of
neurons (Angevine, '65; Sidman, '70). By combining the data

from these two studies, we can reconstruct the fate of neuroglia from precursor cell to mature macroglia.

We have used the optic nerve for our studies of glial development since only glial precursors are present in the nerve rather than a combination of undifferentiated neuronal and glial cells. It is also a small and an easily isolated tract so that quantitative studies may be easily performed.

The development of this nerve is similar to other regions of the brain in that it consists initially of a central canal lined by ventricular cells. These ventricular cells are presumably the source of all the macroglia contained within the adult nerve. In the rat and the mouse, the animals upon which our data is based, the optic canal becomes obliterated about 15 to 17 days of gestation. The nerve at this time consists of axons of retinal ganglion cells and neuroglia. While most of the cells appear undifferentiated using routine electron microscopy, our radiographic studies indicate that a few astrocytes have already completed their final cell division (Skoff et al '76b). Most of the astroglia, though, are not generated until the first week of postnatal life. Formation of astrocytes declines after the first week and now oligodendrocytes begin their final cell division in large numbers. Their maximum period of production is between 5 and 10 days after birth and by 16 days has reached background levels.

The precursor cells that give rise to astrocytes and oligodendrocytes formed during postnatal development can be identified by injecting ^{3}H-thymidine one hour prior to sacrifice. One hour after an injection of radioactive thymidine, only those cells about to enter mitosis are labelled since they are still in the DNA synthetic phase or have just entered the G_2 phase which immediately precedes cell division (Baserga, '65). Light microscopic autoradiograms of nerves and spinal cords prepared from rat and mice sacrificed within an hour after an injection reveal labelled cells that are small and quite different in morphology from mature macroglia (see Figs. in Skoff, '80) and might be classified as undifferentiated glioblasts. However, the electron microscopic autoradiograms provide much more information about the nature of the proliferating cells. After birth most of the labelled cells can be classified as immature astroglia or oligodendroglia rather than undifferentiated glioblasts (Skoff, '76a). It is important to stress that the labelled cells differ in many respects from mature astroglia and oligodendroglia. Still, it is possible to reconstruct the sequence of differentiation from immature to mature cells by recognizing features of more differentiated cells in the less differentiated forms. Immature glia differ from mature cells not so much in the type of organelles they contain but more so in regards to their relative number and distribution within the cytoplasm. As an example, mature oligodendroglia are characterized by fascicles of microtubules in their processes and cytoplasm but in immature oligodendroglia, they occur singly and are often arranged at various angles to one another. However, as young astroglia often contain clusters of microtubules, the presence or absence of this organelle in a particular cell type should not be used as the only criterion. Other features helpful in the identification of immature oligodendroglia include an electron dense matrix and an abundance of mitochondria and cisternae of the Golgi apparatus. These organelles gradually come to occupy less volume in the mature cell but they still appear more prominent than in astroglia and microglia. A detailed discussion of the identification of differentiating glia is presented in the following papers (Skoff et al., '76a, b and Skoff, '80). The labelled cell illustrated in this paper (Fig. 1) is typical of many of the labelled oligodendroblasts observed in development except that the density of this cell is darker and more akin to that of the mature form.

The results of our autoradiographic studies indicate that the astrocytes and oligodendrocytes formed during postnatal development arise primarily from astroblasts and oligodendroblasts rather than undifferentiated glioblasts. Postnatally, then, macroglial cells arise from two cell lines rather than from a multipotential glial cell. The low percentage of labelled microglial cells (2%) in the optic nerve indicates that this cell type is not a major source of glia nor does it function as a multipotential cell.

PROLIFERATION OF OLIGODENDROGLIAL CELLS IN JIMPY MICE

The information obtained about the morphology and differentiation of neuroglia in normal animals provides the basis for studying myelinogenesis and gliogenesis in experimental models of human disease and in neurological

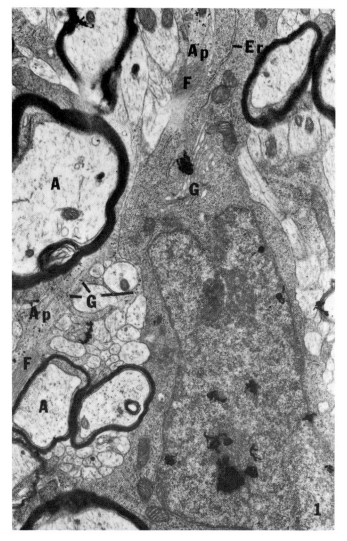

Fig. 1. This electron microscopic autoradiogram shows silver grains overlying the nucleus of an oligodendroblast. This picture is from the spinal cord of a 7 day old normal animal. The cytoplasm of this cell is packed with free ribosomes contained in an electron dense matrix. Contrast the cytoplasmic density of this cell with axoplasm (A) and astrocytic processes (Ap). The astrocyte processes are characterized by filaments (F) and glycogen particles (G). Mitochondria, cisterns of Golgi apparatus (G) and thin strands of rough endoplasmic reticulum (ER) are also present in the cytoplasm. x18,000.

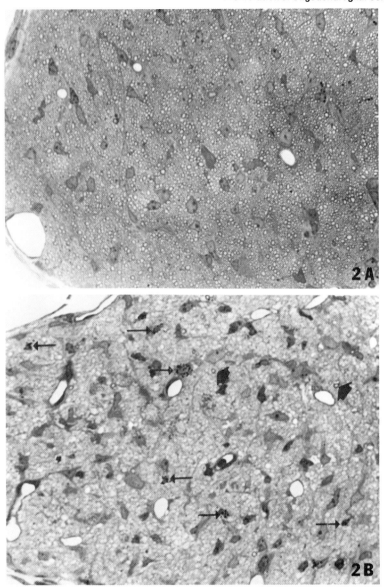

Fig. 2. Light microscopic autoradiograms of optic nerves
from 20 day old mice. A normal, control nerve is shown in
2A and a Jimpy in 2B. The animals were sacrificed one hour
after an injection of ^{3}H-thymidine. Note the paucity of
myelin sheaths in the mutant (arrowheads). Labelled cells
are absent or rarely observed in normal animals at this age
but they are common in the affected animals (arrows). x2,100.

mutants. We have recently examined cell proliferation in the Jimpy mouse, a mutant that has almost no myelin in the CNS (Sidman et al., '64; Meier et al., '74). The mutation is sex-linked, recessive and fatal between 20 and 30 days after birth (Phillips, '54). The peripheral nervous system (PNS) does not appear to be affected by the mutation (although no quantitative studies of myelin content have been made). The myelin deficit is due to the failure of the oligodendrocytes to elaborate myelin in substantial amounts rather than to a subsequent degeneration of the myelin sheath (Farkas-Bargeton et al., '72; Meier et al., '74). The underlying cause of the myelin deficiency has not been determined although there have been numerous morphological and biochemical studies (e.g., Nusbaum et al., '69; Mandel et al., '72; Neskovic et al., '72; Meier et al., '74). A reduction in the number of oligodendrocytes is one factor that could contribute to the myelin deficiency and we have shown in a previous electron microscopic study that their number is reduced about 50% (Skoff, '76). This reduction is certainly one of the elements responsible for the paucity of the myelin but does not explain its virtual absence. Neither is the cause of the oligodendrocyte reduction apparent. This could be due to a variety of causes including cell death or decreased cell proliferation.

We have recently compared the rates of cell proliferation and the morphology of the dividing cells in the affected males with normal, male littermates at various stages of development. Four different developmental stages were examined (4, 7-9, 15-18 and 20-22 days after birth). At each stage at least five normal and five Jimpy animals were analyzed. For each animal, a minimum of two different sections were quantitated from the spinal cord and both sides of the optic nerve. The animals were given a single injection of ^{3}H-thymidine and then sacrificed one hour later (see Skoff et al., '76a for details). The mitotic index was calculated by determining the percentage of labelled cells in complete transverse sections of the optic nerve and in the white matter of the spinal cord. Up to 9 days after birth, the mitotic index is the same for both normals and mutants but by 16 days a significant change takes place. Around 16 days after birth, cell proliferation in normal mice slows to background levels but continues at a high rate in the mutants. In the 15-18 day old animals, the mitotic index is 1.5 for normal mice and 5.7 for the mutants. At 20 days after birth, the mitotic index continues to decline for normals (0.42) but remains quite high (3.20) for the

Jimpys (Fig. 2). The high mitotic index in the mutants should produce a major increase in the total number of glia but quantitation of their numbers does not reveal much of a change. At 20-22 days of age, the total glial cell number is increased by 10% in the spinal cord and reduced by 10% in the optic nerve. The fact that the total number of cells is not in line with the mitotic index indicates that the thymidine labelled cells must either be dividing and then dying, incorporating thymidine without subsequent cell division or dividing over an abnormally long cell cycle. Cell death is probably one of the factors since our light microscopic observations reveal numerous moribund cells in the mutants.

Analysis of electron microscopic autoradiograms from the normals and mutants at different stages of development provide additional information about the proliferative capabilities of oligodendrocytes. Between 4 and 10 days of development, the same type of cells are labelled in the mutants as in the normal animals (i.e., astroblasts, oligodendroblasts and microglia). The oligodendroblasts, though, have less cytoplasm and appear less differentiated than their normal counterparts. From 16 to 22 days after birth, about 70% of the labelled cells in the Jimpy mouse can be classified as oligodendroblasts (Fig. 3) or glioblasts. These glioblasts appear to be in the **oligodendrocyte line but have too few characteristic** features for a positive identification. The remainder of the labelled cells can be classified as microglia (30%) (Fig. 4) or astrocytes (5-10%). Although the astrocytes show a dramatic increase in their processes (Skoff, '76), it is surprising that they are not hyperplastic even at the later stages of development. Our electron microscopic autoradiographic data shows that oligodendroglial cells are capable of incorporating tritiated thymidine much like their counterparts in normal animals. They continue to become labelled beyond their normal period of proliferation. Therefore, the paucity of oligodendroglial cells in the mutants cannot be accounted for by a decrease in cell proliferation. A more likely explanation is that they continue to incorporate thymidine but then fail to complete their normal course of differentiation. The failure of the cells to make myelin may be due to some factor (either intrinsic or extrinsic) that affects their division and differentiation rather than to a defect in the synthesis of myelin components. Continued autoradiographic investigations

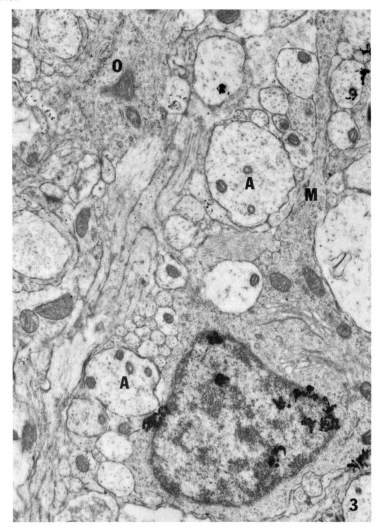

Fig. 3. This labelled oligodendroblast is from the spinal cord of a 16 day old Jimpy. Note the absence of myelin sheaths around the axons (A). This oligodendroblast contains the same organelles as the cell in Fig. 2 but the matrix is considerably less dense. The cytoplasm of this cell has a long process that contains a bundle of microtubules (M). A portion of another oligodendrocyte (O) may be compared to the labelled cell and to astrocytic processes which contain filaments and glycogen. The nucleus of this cell and the immature oligodendrocyte shown in Fig. 2 is eccentrically located, a feature frequently seen in immature cells of this line. x18,000.

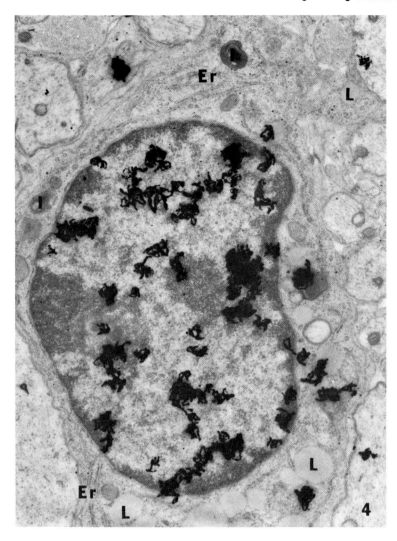

Fig. 4. A labelled microglial cell from the spinal cord of a 16 day old mutant. The cytoplasm is characterized by numerous lipid droplets (L), membranous inclusions (I), and long, thin strands of rough endoplasmic reticulum (ER). The density of this cell is intermediate to astrocytes and oligodendrocytes. The cytoplasm of these cells contain fewer microtubules, ribosomes, and cisternae of the Golgi apparatus in comparison to oligodendroglia. x17,000.

will allow us to determine the length of their cell cycle,
the extent of cell death and if these cells proliferate
without exiting from the cell cycle.

This work was supported by a U.S.P.H.S. Grant (NS15338) and
a Basil O'Connor Grant from the National Foundation-March of
Dimes.

Angevine JB Jr (1965). Time of neuron origin in the
   hippocampal region An autoradiographic study in the mouse.
   Expt Neurol Suppl 2,13:1-70.
Baserga R (1965). The relationship of the cell cycle to
   tumor growth and control of cell division: A review.
   Cancer Res 25:581-595.
Farkas-Bargeton E, Robain O, Mandel P (1972). Abnormal glial
   maturation in the white matter in Jimpy mice An optical
   study. Acta neuropath (Berl) 21:272-281.
Mandel P, Nussbaum JL, Neskovic NM, Sarlieve LL, Kurihara T
   (1972). Regulation of myelinogenesis. In Weber G (ed):
   "Advances in Enzyme Regulation," Oxford: Pergamon, vol 10,
   p 101-118.
Meier C, Herschkowitz N, Bischoff A (1974). Morphological
   and biochemical observations in the Jimpy spinal cord.
   Acta Neuropath 27:349-362.
Neskovic NM, Sarlieve LL, Mandel P (1972). Biosynthesis of
   glycolipids in myelin deficient mutants: Brain glycosyl
   transferase in jimpy and quaking mice. Brain Res 42:147-157.
Nussbaum JL, Neskovic P, Mandel P (1969). A study of lipid
   components in brain of the "jimpy" mouse, a mutant with
   myelin deficiency. J Neurochem 16:927-934.
Phillips DE (1973). An electron microscopic study of
   macroglia and microglia in the lateral funiculus of the
   developing spinal cord in the fetal monkey. Z Zellforsch
   140:145-167.
Phillips RJS (1954). Jimpy, a new totally sex-linked gene in
   the house mouse. Zeit fur indukt Abstammungs und
   Vererbungslehre 86:322-326.
Sidman RL (1970). Autoradiographic methods and principles
   for study of the nervous system with thymidine-H^3. In
   Nauta WJH, Ebbesson SOE (eds): "Contemporary Research
   Methods in Neuroanatomy," New York: Springer-Verlag,
   p 252-274.
Sidman RL, Dickie MM, Appel SH (1964). Mutant mice (quaking
   and jimpy) with deficient myelination in the central
   nervous system. Science 144:309-311.

Skoff RP (1976). Myelin deficit in the Jimpy mouse may be due to cellular abnormalities in astroglia. Nature 264: 560-562.

Skoff RP (1980). Neuroglia: a reevaluation of their origin and development. In Fujita S (ed): "Cytogenesis and Cellular Pathology of Neuroglia and Microglia," Stuttgart: Springer.

Skoff RP, Price DL, Stocks A (1976a). Electron microscopic autoradiographic studies of gliogenesis in rat optic nerve I Cell proliferation. J Comp Neurol 169:291-312.

Skoff RP, Price DL, Stocks A (1976b). Electron microscopic autoradiographic studies of gliogenesis in rat optic nerve II Time of origin. J Comp Neurol 169:313-333.

Sturrock RR (1974). Histogenesis of the anterior limb of the anterior commissure of the mouse brain III An electron microscopic study of gliogenesis. J Anat 117:1:37-53.

Vaughn JE (1969). An electron microscopic analysis of gliogenesis in rat optic nerves. Z Zellforsch 94:293-324.

Eleventh International Congress of Anatomy:
Glial and Neuronal Cell Biology, pages 105 – 109
© 1981 Alan R. Liss, Inc., 150 Fifth Avenue, New York, NY 10011

Remyelination in the CNS

W.F. Blakemore

Department of Clinical Veterinary
Medicine, Madingley Road,
Cambridge, CB3 OES
Our understanding of remyelination in the central nervous
system has changed dramatically in the last 10 years; however
we are still a long way from fully understanding the process
and, in particular, factors which inhibit it. I will first
examine some known facts about the process and then consider
some observations which may necessitate a re-evaluation of
our thinking about diseases such as multiple sclerosis.

Observations on cuprizone induced demyelination in the
mouse have illustrated three basic facts about remyelination.
In the cuprizone model the superior cerebellar peduncle can be
reliably demyelinated allowing features of remyelinated sheaths
to be established (Blakemore, 1973 a & b).When myelin sheath
thickness is related to axon diameter it can be shown that
remyelinated sheaths never return to the normal relationship;
they are always thinner than normal (Blakemore, 1974). When
repair is complete it is difficult or impossible to
distinguish areas of remyelination from normal white matter by
light microscopy, even using plastic sections. Therefore,
remyelination cannot be easily detected in human material
using standard techniques. For this reason the inherent
ability of the human C.N.S. to remyelinate has probably been
underestimated.

In the cuprizone system demyelination follows degeneration
of oligodendrocytes (Blakemore, 1971) and these cells are
replaced by mitosis from a yet undetermined cell type (Ludwin,
1978, 1979). This cell may be an oligodendrocyte or an
uncommitted stem cell (Ludwin, 1979). Oligodendrocyte
replacement has also been indirectly demonstrated in the rat

and cat spinal cord using local injections of lysolecithin as
the method for oligodendrocyte destruction (Blakemore, 1976,
Blakemore et al 1977). A further observation made on the
cuprizone model is that little, if any, remyelination occurs
if the animals are maintained on the cuprizone diet although
oligodendrocytes can be seen among the demyelinated axons
(Blakemore, 1973a). This separation of cell replacement and
remyelination (Blakemore, 1979) will be referred to again
later.

Although the cuprizone lesion has certain advantages its
usefulness as a model system is limited as it is not easy to
carry out physiological studies, examine nerve fibres in
longitudinal section, or undertake multiple experimentation.
More favourable lesions can be made using injections of small
volumes of gliotoxic chemicals into the spinal cord. These
can be positioned so that physiological and morphological
studies can be facilitated and they also open up the
possibility of secondary experimentation on the focal areas of
demyelination so produced.

Using injections of lysolecithin in the cat spinal cord
it has been shown that the morphological events of
demyelination and remyelination relate well to the electrophysiological demonstration of block and restoration of nerve
conduction (Smith et al 1979). These studies showed that
association of ensheathing cells with axons commenced 7 days
after initiation of demyelination and some remyelination with
restoration of conduction had occurred by 14 days. After 81
days no further improvement in conduction occurred by which
time the refractory period of transmission was normal. These
observations, taken with those on the cuprizone model indicate
that under favourable conditions remyelination rapidly follows
demyelination and proceeds to completion over a short period
of time. This situation differs from that found in multiple
sclerosis where areas of demyelination persist. It is
therefore pertinent to examine situations in which the
remyelination process does not proceed rapidly to completion.

If one makes focal demyelinating lesions in the rabbit
spinal cord using lysolecithin, demyelination results but
unlike similar lesions in the rat and cat (Blakemore, 1976,
Blakemore et al 1977), not all the axons are remyelinated
(Blakemore, 1978). Rather some are remyelinated, those near
the edge of the lesion, while axons in the centre of the lesion
remain demyelinated for up to six months. The axons

remyelinated by oligodendrocytes lie near to normal tissue and
the area contains a good astrocytic presence, while the axons
that remain demyelinated lie in an area containing few
astrocytic processes and myelin debris persists in the
extracellular space. Oligodendrocytes however, are present
and in some cases small oligodendrocyte processes relate to the
axons but this association does not progress to myelination.
Thus oligodendrocytes and demyelinated axons are present, but
remyelination is not taking place. The difference between the
two zones is not the presence or absence of oligodendrocytes,
rather it is an absence of astrocytes and presence of myelin
debris in the area where remyelination is not occurring. A
similar situation exists following local injection of
6-aminonicotinamide (6-AN) into the rat spinal cord (Blakemore,
1975).

Following 6-AN injections glial cells are destroyed, both
oligodendrocytes and astrocytes; however, astrocytes are
destroyed over a larger area than oligodendrocytes. As a
direct result of the astrocyte destruction Schwann cells invade
the spinal cord and myelinate nearly all the demyelinated
axons (Blakemore, 1979), the only axons remyelinated by
oligodendrocytes lie close to normal tissue around the edge of
the lesion. The failure of oligodendrocytes to remyelinate
axons, as would happen if the demyelination had been caused
by lysolecithin cannot be explained by a lack of these cells
as groups of oligodendrocytes can be found near to demyelinated
axons at intermediate times. Rather as in the rabbit
lysolecithin lesions, the reason may be the lack of astrocytes
in the area containing the demyelinated axons. That
myelinating cells and signalling axons are insufficient for
myelination to occur has been demonstrated for Schwann cells in
tissue culture by the Bunges (Bunge and Bunge, 1978). They
consider that the third element in that system is collagen;
indicating the need for a third factor in the myelination
process. In the C.N.S. the third factor may well be
astrocytes as indicated by the 6-AN and rabbit lysolecithin
experiments (Blakemore, 1975, 1978).

Thus it appears that the presence of oligodendrocytes and
axons signalling ensheathment, does not ensure remyelination
will occur. I have discussed the possible involvement of
astrocytes in this process and would now like to turn to
evidence which indicates that even in the presence of this
cell remyelination will not occur if there is persistence of
the demyelinating stimulus. This was shown to be the case

with cuprizone, where the replacement oligodendrocytes only
myelinated when the animals were taken off the cuprizone diet.
The same phenomenon has been more elegantly demonstrated in
tissue culture by Bornstein and Raine (Bornstein and Raine,
1970, Raine and Bornstein, 1970). Myelinated tissue cultures
can be demyelinated by 25% myelinotoxic serum obtained from
animals with acute E.A.E. When the culture is washed
remyelination occurs. If however, the serum remains in the
culture medium the culture remains demyelinated. This applies
even if the concentration of myelinotoxic serum is reduced
below a level which can induce demyelination. Thus
demyelinating factors can inhibit myelination and remyelination
even when they fall below a level capable of initiating
demyelination. The repair in chronic E.A.E. which follows
desensitisation suggests a similar association between
demyelination and inhibited repair in vivo (Raine et al, 1978a,
1978b).

In conclusion, it now seems likely that the demyelinated
lesions of M.S. are not a reflection of the inability of the
human C.N.S. to carry out remyelination, rather they could be
an integral part of the pathogenesis of this disease. That
similar lesions in experimental animals can be reversed
offers hope to M.S. patients.

References

Blakemore WF (1971). Observations on oligodendrocyte
degeneration, the resolution of status spongiosus and
remyelination in cuprizone intoxication in mice. J
neurocytol 1:413.

Blakemore WF (1973a). Demyelination of the superior cerebellar
perduncle in the mouse induced by cuprizone. J neurol Sci
20:63.

Blakemore WF (1973b). Remyelination of the superior cerebellar
peduncle in the mouse following demyelination induced by
feeding cuprizone. J neurol Sci 20:73.

Blakemore WF (1974). Pattern of remyelination in the CNS.
Nature 249:577.

Blakemore WF (1975). Remyelination by Schwann cells of axons
demyelinated by intraspinal injections of
6-aminonicotinamide. J neurocytol 4:475.

Blakemore WF (1976). Invasion of Schwann cells into the spinal
cord of the rat following local injections of lysolecithin.
J neuropath appl neurobiol 2:21.

Blakemore WF (1978). Observations on remyelination in the rabbit spinal cord following demyelination induced by lysolecithin. J neuropath appl neurobiol 4:47

Blakemore WF (1979). Remyelination in the CNS. In Progress in Neurological Research ed PO Behan and F Clifford Rose Pittman Bath p 12.

Blakemore WF, Eames RA, Smith KJ McDonald WI (1977). Remyelination in the spinal cord of the cat following intraspinal injections of lysolecithin. J neurol Sci 33:31

Bornstein MB Raine CS (1970). Experimental allergic encephalomyelitis: antiserum inhibition of myelination in vitro. Lab Invest 23:536.

Bunge RP Bunge MB (1978). Evidence that a contact with commective tissue matrix is required for normal interaction between Schwann cells and nerve fibres. J cell Biol 78:943.

Ludwin SK (1979). An autoradiographic study of cellular proliferation in remyelination of the central nervous system. Amer J Path 95:683.

Ludwin SK (1978). Central nervous system demyelination and remyelination in the mouse: an ultrastructural study of cuprizone toxicity. Lab Invest 39:597.

Raine CS Bornstein MB (1970). Experimental allergic encephalomyelitis: an ultrastructural study of experimental demyelination in vitro. J neuropath exp neurol 29:552.

Raine CS, Traugott U Stone SH (1978a). Suppression of chronic allergic encephalomyelitis: relevance to multiple sclerosis. Science 201:445.

Raine CS, Traugott U Stone SH (1978b). Chronic relapsing experimental allergic encephalomyelitis: CNS plaque development in unsuppressed and suppressed animals. Acta neuropath 43:43.

Smith KJ, Blakemore WF McDonald WI (1979). Central remyelination restores secure conduction. Nature 280:395.

STRUCTURE AND FUNCTION
OF MICROGLIA

Eleventh International Congress of Anatomy:
Glial and Neuronal Cell Biology, pages 113–124
© 1981 Alan R. Liss, Inc., 150 Fifth Avenue, New York, NY 10011

MICROGLIA, MONOCYTES, AND MACROPHAGES[1]

Erle K. Adrian, Jr. and Robert L. Schelper

Departments of Anatomy and Pathology
The University of Texas Health Science Center
at San Antonio, San Antonio, Texas, U. S. A.

The relationships of microglia and monocytes to each other and to macrophages have been the subjects of many investigations (reviewed by Russell, 1962; Privat, 1975; Oehmichen, 1978). The earliest investigators of this problem believed that brain macrophages were derived from leucocytes. Later investigators thought they were derived from glial cells or from cells associated with vessels, such as pericytes or adventitial cells, or from microglia, or from both endogenous and exogenous sources. With the advent of labeling techniques using tritiated thymidine (^{3}H-TdR), interest again shifted to a hematogenous source, in particular the blood monocyte, as the cell type from which most or all CNS macrophages were derived (Konigsmark and Sidman, 1963; Kitamura *et al.*, 1972). Other investigators, in particular Vaughn and coworkers (Vaughn and Peters, 1968; Vaughn *et al.*, 1970), postulated a third type of glial cell that was morphologically similar to microglia, but of neuroectodermal origin, as the cell of origin of brain macrophages. Recently, there has been a shift to the concept of a graded response from both endogenous and exogenous sources (Vaughn and Skoff, 1972).

Much of the modern investigative work which supports a hematogenous source for some or all brain macrophages is based on the use of ^{3}H-TdR as a pulse label for cells in DNA synthesis. Following injection, ^{3}H-TdR is available for incorporation into DNA for a period of an hour or less (Blenkinsopp, 1968). Repeated injections of ^{3}H-TdR given to

1 Supported by USPHS Grant NS 08949

mice with the last injection 16 to 24 hours before nervous
tissue injury have resulted in the presence of many labeled
macrophages, microglial cells, and fibroblasts in the injured
tissue (Adrian et al., 1978). Since the labeled thymidine
was not believed to be available to label cells proliferating
in response to injury, the hypothesis was advanced that these
reactive cells were derived from circulating blood mononuclear cells which were labeled in the hematopoietic tissues
at the time of ^{3}H-TdR injection (Adrian and Walker, 1962;
Walker, 1963; Konigsmark and Sidman, 1963). Most of the
experiments that will be discussed in this presentation were
designed to test this hypothesis or the alternative hypothesis that labeled DNA precursor material, which can label
intrinsic cells proliferating in response to the injury,
becomes available many hours after ^{3}H-TdR injection.

Our principal research interest has not been directly
concerned with CNS macrophages per se, but rather has been
to identify the various populations of cells that react to
nervous tissue injury by synthesizing DNA and dividing and
to study the functional role of these cells in repair and
regeneration of nervous tissue. In particular we have
attempted to determine the contribution of blood mononuclear
cells to the proliferative response to stab wounds of the
spinal cord and to the central proliferative response to
peripheral nerve injury.

Many of the studies concerning the origin of the
cells that take part in the central reaction to peripheral
nerve injury have presented data that appear to be in direct
conflict. The majority of investigators have concluded that
the reactive cells are endogenous microglia (for example,
Sjöstrand, 1971). However, a number of independent studies
using either the injection of labeled blood mononuclear cells
(Roessman and Friede, 1968) or multiple injections of ^{3}H-TdR
prior to nerve injury (Adrian and Smothermon, 1970; Fujita
and Kitamura, 1976; Young, 1977a,b; Adrian et al., 1978)
have demonstrated the presence of labeled cells, which have
the appearance of reactive microglia, in the nuclei of
damaged peripheral nerves, again suggesting that these cells
are derived from circulating blood mononuclear cells. These
studies for the most part have not been confirmed by other
techniques of labeling cells derived from the blood
(Stenwig, 1972; Oehmichen and Torvik, 1976), although Persson
et al. (1978) did find that antiserum to rat peritoneal

macrophages reacted with perineuronal microglial cells following facial nerve transection.

In both direct invasive trauma to the spinal cord (Adrian and Williams, 1973), and in indirect injuries to the CNS, such as a peripheral nerve transection (Kerns and Hinsman, 1973a, b), the majority of the proliferating cells found later in the central nervous system have ultrastructural features of microglia (Mori and Leblond, 1969). In order to determine if such cells could be derived from circulating blood mononuclear cells, we gave mice repeated injections of ^{3}H-TdR with the last injection at least 16 hours before either a stab wound to the spinal cord (Adrian *et al.*, 1978) or transection of the hypoglossal nerve. About half of the labeled cells in the injured spinal cords and virtually all the labeled cells in the nuclei of the injured nerves had nuclei with peripheral heterochromatin, dark cytoplasm with long cisterns of granular endoplasmic reticulum and other ultrastructural features of microglia. Since uninjured nervous tissue has only a small number of labeled cells with this experimental protocol, two possible explanations may be given for the origin of these labeled cells. The first is that if ^{3}H-TdR is truly a pulse label available for incorporation into DNA for only a short time following its injection, with no subsequent reappearance in the systemic circulation, then all or most of the labeled cells in the injured tissue must be blood derived mononuclear leucocytes, as there was no other reservoir of labeled cells available to the nervous tissue. In that case the finding of a large number of labeled microglial cells indicates that microglia are derived from hematogenous cells. On the other hand, the second possible explanation for these labeled cells is that if there was a significant amount of reutilization of the labeled thymidine, then some and possibly all of the labeled cells found outside of vessels might be intrinsic nervous tissue cells proliferating in response to the injury.

Since the monocyte is the blood mononuclear cell that has most often been associated with reactive microglia and CNS macrophages, we decided next to test the hypothesis that the reactive microglia found in the injured spinal cord and the nucleus of the injured hypoglossal nerve are derived from blood monocytes (Schelper and Adrian, in press). Monocytes and cells in the monocytic series have been shown to contain marked diffuse cytoplasmic activity of nonspecific esterase (NSE) (Schmalzl and Braunsteiner, 1970). If reactive microglia and spinal cord macrophages are derived from monocytes, then it should be possible to demonstrate NaF sensitive NSE in their cytoplasm. Absence of this enzyme in microglia should rule out the monocyte as a precursor to that cell type.

Adult female mice were each given three injections of ^{3}H-TdR over an eight hour period. They were then randomly divided into three groups of eight, one group receiving spinal cord stab wounds, one group receiving left hypoglossal nerve transection, and one group left as uninjured controls. At 2, 4, 8, or 16 days after injury pairs of mice from each group were anesthetized and killed by intracardiac perfusion of formal-calcium fixative. After removal of the brainstem or spinal cord, postfixation in formal calcium, and soaking in 0.88M sucrose in 0.9% gum arabic for 48-72 hours, frozen sections were cut and stained for NaF sensitive NSE activity as described by Shnitka and Seligman (1961). These sections were then processed for radioautography. After development, sections of medulla or spinal cord were selected at random for study. Fifty 100X fields were scanned on each spinal cord section, and the number of cells in each of the following categories was recorded: labeled and having NaF sensitive NSE activity, labeled and having no NaF sensitive NSE activity, and unlabeled and having NaF sensitive NSE activity. The results are summarized in Fig. 1. The uninjured controls had few labeled cells, none of which had any NaF sensitive NSE activity. In the injured animals the number of such labeled cells without NSE activity was 10 to 30 times greater than the number in the controls. In addition, every injured animal had many labeled and unlabeled cells containing NaF-sensitive NSE, which were mainly in the wound. About 7% of the total number of labeled cells had NaF-sensitive NSE. The rest of the labeled cells were found in small numbers in the neuropil away from the area of injury and were concentrated heavily in the area of injury. Such cells always far outnumbered the cells with NaF sensitive NSE activity.

Several randomly selected sections containing both hypoglossal nuclei were examined from each uninjured control and from each mouse subjected to hypoglossal axotomy. In the injured animals at each time interval, from nine to forty labeled cells per section were found in the nucleus of the

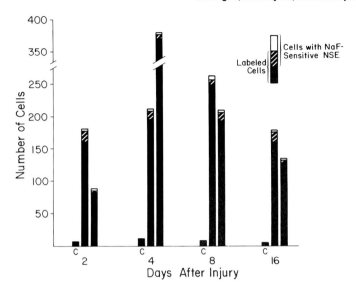

Fig. 1. Number of cells in 50 100X fields of spinal cord having a radioactive label and/or sodium fluoride sensitive non-specific esterase activity. Three injections of ^{3}H-TdR on the day before injury. Each bar represents one animal. C is uninjured control.

injured nerve and from one to six labeled cells were found in the contralateral nucleus. The uninjured controls never had more than one labeled cell per section in either hypoglossal nucleus. No cells with NaF sensitive NSE activity were found in any tissue section at any time interval.

Therefore, the spinal cord wounds contained labeled cells with NaF sensitive NSE activity which were presumably monocytes or macrophages. A much larger number of labeled cells were present that did not have NaF sensitive NSE activity. These cells may have been some other type of blood mononuclear cell, such as a lymphocyte, or they may have been intrinsic non-neuronal cells that were labeled by reutilization of ^{3}H-TdR. All of the labeled cells in the hypoglossal nuclei lacked NaF sensitive NSE activity, and therefore, were not derived from monocytes. Since these cells have previously been shown to have the ultrastructure of reactive microglia,

these findings do not support the hypothesis that microglia
are identical with or derived from blood monocytes. Rather,
they may have been derived from some other type of blood
mononuclear cell, or they have become labeled by reutilization
of ^{3}H-TdR.

To test for the possibility of ^{3}H-TdR reutilization by
intrinsic cells proliferating in response to nervous tissue
injury as an explanation for the labeled cells observed in
the previous experiment that did not have NaF sensitive NSE
activity, the experiment was repeated using the thymidine
analogue ^{125}I-5-iodo-2'-deoxyuridine (^{125}I-UdR) to label the
hematopoietic tissues prior to spinal cord stab wounds and
transection of the hypoglossal nerve (Schelper and Adrian,
in press). Since ^{125}I-UdR is specifically incorporated into
DNA but with a much lower rate of reutilization than ^{3}H-TdR
(Feinendegen *et al.*, 1973), comparison of the numbers and
types of labeled cells found using ^{125}I-UdR with those found
using ^{3}H-TdR should reveal how much, if any, that labeling of
proliferating intrinsic cells by reutilization of ^{3}H-TdR was
contributing to the population of labeled cells previously
observed in the injured tissues. The results of this experiment are summarized in Fig. 2.

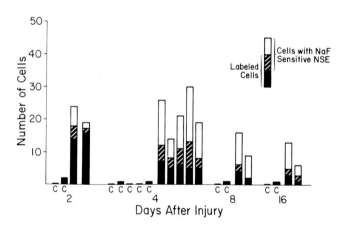

Fig. 2. Number of cells in 50 100X fields of spinal cord
having a radioactive label and/or sodium fluoride sensitive
non-specific esterase activity. Three injections of
[125]I-UdR on the day before injury. Each bar represents one
animal. C is uninjured control.

As in the experiment in which ^{3}H-TdR was injected prior to injury, there were many more labeled cells in the injured spinal cords than in uninjured controls; however, the total number of such labeled cells was much less than in the earlier experiment. A much higher percentage of the labeled cells had NaF-sensitive NSE activity. This finding is consistent with reutilization of ^{3}H-TdR by proliferating intrinsic cells as the explanation for the large number of labeled cells not having NaF sensitive NSE when ^{3}H-TdR was injected before injury. However, the majority of the ^{125}I-UdR labeled cells in this experiment also had no NSE activity and therefore may be non-monocytic hematogenous cells.

When we examined the sections of brainstem containing the hypoglossal nuclei, no more than one labeled cell was found in any section and many sections had no labeled cells. The occasional labeled cell was not restricted to the side of injury. Since there was no difference in the number of labeled cells found in the nucleus of the injured nerve and in the hypoglossal nucleus of uninjured controls, the hypothesis that the ^{3}H-TdR labeled microglia observed in the preceding experiments were labeled by ^{3}H-TdR reutilization is strongly supported by this experiment.

To rule out a possible inhibition of the proliferative response to peripheral nerve injury by ^{125}I-UdR, counts of the non-neuronal, non-vascular cells in each hypoglossal nucleus were made. These counts revealed about a 25% increase in the number of such cells in the nucleus of the injured nerve, showing that the injections of ^{125}I-UdR before injury did not inhibit the proliferation of reactive non-neuronal cells. To rule out the possibility that these proliferating cells were unable to use ^{125}I-UdR in DNA synthesis, ^{125}I-UdR was given on the fourth day after hypoglossal nerve transection, and many labeled cells were found in the nuclei of the injured nerves. When ^{3}H-TdR and ^{125}I-UdR were injected simultaneously on the day before hypoglossal nerve injury with sacrifice four days after injury many labeled cells were found in the nuclei of the injured nerves, just as when ^{3}H-TdR alone had been used. Therefore, ^{125}I-UdR had no inhibitory effect on microglial proliferation or the uptake of ^{3}H-TdR following hypoglossal nerve injury. Finally, to rule out the possibility that the inefficient incorporation of ^{125}I-UdR resulted in too few labeled blood mononuclear cells in the peripheral blood to allow them to be detected in the hypoglossal nucleus, six mice were injected with ^{125}I-UdR every five hours for a total of twelve injections so that the number of labeled large mononuclear cells in the peripheral blood exceeded 40% at the time of injury. The population of non-neuronal, non-vascular cells increased on the side of injury as before; however, none of these cells was labeled. Therefore, these reactive cells are not derived from the population of large mononuclear leucocytes labeled with ^{125}I-UdR, and the absence of labeled cells in the nucleus of the injured nerve cannot be attributed to an insufficient degree of labeling of this cell population (Schelper and Adrian, in press).

The experiments in this series have ruled out all hypotheses that we could think of, other than ^{3}H-TdR reutilization, that could explain the presence of labeled cells in the nucleus of the injured hypoglossal nerve when ^{3}H-TdR was given before injury and their absence when ^{125}I-UdR was given before injury. Since there was no local destruction of labeled cells in the hypoglossal nucleus or elsewhere in the brain, these results imply systemic availability of ^{3}H-TdR at periods much greater than the one hour or less after injection that has been reported by numerous authors. This finding has a direct and important bearing on the interpretation of the results of many long-term studies of cell migration and transformation using ^{3}H-TdR. Work that has recently been completed in our laboratory has confirmed the presence of a systemically available DNA precursor in the blood between 2 and 9 days after injection of ^{3}H-TdR (Williams and Adrian, 1978, 1980).

To test the hypothesis that the cells that proliferate in the hypoglossal nucleus following hypoglossal axotomy are derived exclusively from intrinsic cells of the nervous tissue, we decided to use a very different labeling procedure from those that have been discussed thus far. In this experiment we decided to label the glial population while leaving the hematogenous cells unlabeled, which is exactly the reverse of the previous experiments. Similar experiments have been done previously by Smith and Walker (1967), Asbury (1970), and Murray and Walker (1973). Daily injections of 5μCi of ^{3}H-TdR were given to 14 A/J mice during the first 10 days of postnatal life. By 20 weeks of age peripheral blood smears were essentially free of labeled leucocytes, while a large proportion of the glial and endothelial population was labeled. At 20 weeks of age, seven of these mice were anesthetized and the left hypoglossal nerve of each was cut.

Four days later all 14 mice were anesthetized and sacrificed by intracardiac perfusion of fixative. Sections of medulla containing the hypoglossal nuclei were processed for radio-autography, and random sections from each animal from the region of the obex were chosen for study. All non-neuronal cells in a 0.16 mm^2 area enclosing each hypoglossal nucleus were observed at 100X and classified as vascular cells (endothelial cells and pericytes), perineuronal satellites, or other non-neuronal cells. Each cell was also examined for the presence of a radioactive label. There was no significant difference between the nuclei of the injured nerves and control nuclei in the number of labeled or unlabeled vascular cells, labeled perineuronal satellites, or labeled other non-neuronal cells. However, there were about 450% (p<0.001) more unlabeled perineuronal satellites (Fig. 3) in the nucleus of the injured nerve. Since by 20 weeks after ^{3}H-TdR

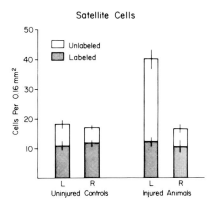

Fig. 3. Number of labeled and unlabeled perineuronal satellite cells in a 0.16 mm^2 area enclosing the hypoglossal nucleus. All animals received 10 daily injections of ^{3}H-TdR during the first 10 days of postnatal life. Half the animals were given left hypoglossal nerve transections at 20 weeks of age. All were sacrificed four days later.

injection there were no labeled circulating blood mononuclear cells, the striking increase in unlabeled cells in the nucleus of the injured nerve could be due to an infiltration of unlabeled mononuclear cells from the blood. However, the experiments already presented have ruled out monocytes and large lymphocytes as a possible source for such an infiltration. Possible sources for these unlabeled reactive cells which have not yet been ruled out include 1) an intrinsic cell type that was not labeled by the series of ^{3}H-TdR injections given during the postnatal period, 2) an intrinsic cell type that was labeled during the postnatal period but which lost that label through repeated divisions during the ensuing 20 weeks, or 3) a population of lymphoid cells not having NaF sensitive NSE which would not have been labeled by the ^{125}I-UdR injections given in the previous experiment.

In conclusion, we have presented evidence that the microglial cells that proliferate in response to nervous tissue injury, and in particular those that divide in response to transection of the hypoglossal nerve, are not derived from blood monocytes. Many of the macrophages found in invasive trauma of the central nervous system are derived from monocytes, but most of the other cells that are found to be labeled in injured nervous tissue when ^{3}H-TdR was injected prior to injury have probably been labeled by reutilization of labeled DNA precursor that becomes available after the injury. Therefore, data from experiments in which ^{3}H-TdR was injected before nervous tissue injury to label circulating blood elements should be interpreted with caution.

REFERENCES

Adrian EK, Smothermon, RD (1970) Leucocytic infiltration into the hypoglossal nucleus labeled with ^{3}H-thymidine injected before transection of the hypoglossal nerve. Anat Rec 166: 99.

Adrian EK, Walker BE (1962). Incorporation of thymidine-H^3 by cells in normal and injured mouse spinal cord. J Neuropath Exp Neurol 21:597.

Adrian EK, Williams, MG (1973) Cell proliferation in injured spinal cord. An electron microscopic study. J Comp Neur 151:1.

Adrian EK, Williams MG, George FC (1978). Fine structure of reactive cells in injured nervous tissue labeled with ^{3}H-thymidine injected before injury. J Comp Neur 180:815.

Asbury AK (1970). The histogenesis of phagocytes during Wallerian degeneration: radioautographic observations. In "VIth Internation Congress of Neuropathology Proceedings," Paris: Masson et Cie, p. 666.

Blenkinsopp WK (1968). Duration of availability of tritiated thymidine following intraperitoneal injection. J Cell Sci 3:91.

Feinendegen LE, Heiniger HG, Friedrich G, Cronkite EP (1973). Difference in reutilization of thymidine in hemopoietic and lymphopoietic tissues of the normal mouse. Cell Tissue Kinet 6:573.

Fujita S, Kitamura T (1976). Origin of brain macrophages and the nature of the microglia. In Zimmerman HM (ed): "Progress in Neuropathology," New York: Grune and Stratton, p. 1.

Kerns JM, Hinsman EJ (1973a). Neuroglial response to sciatic neurectomy. I Light microscopy and autoradiography. J Comp Neur 151:237.

Kerns JM, Hinsman EJ (1973b). Neuroglial response to sciatic neurectomy. II Electron microscopy. J Comp Neur 151:255.

Kitamura T, Hattori H, Fujita S (1972). Autoradiographic studies on histogenesis of brain macrophages in the mouse. J. Neuropath Exp Neurol 31:502.

Konigsmark BW, Sidman RL (1963). Origin of brain macrophages in the mouse. J Neuropath Exp Neurol 22:643.

Mori S, Leblond CP (1969). Identification of microglia in light and electron microscopy. J Comp Neur 135:57.

Murray HM, Walker BE (1973). Comparative study of astrocytes and mononuclear leukocytes reacting to brain trauma in mice. Exp Neurol 41:290.

Oehmichen M (1978). "Mononuclear Phagocytes in the Central Nervous System." Berlin, Heidelberg, New York: Springer-Verlag.

Oehmichen M, Torvik A (1976). The origin of reactive cells in retrograde and Wallerian degeneration. Experiments with intravenous injection of ^{3}H-DFP-labeled macrophages. Cell Tiss Res 173:343.

Persson LI, Rönnbäck L, Rosengren LE (1978). Identification of reactive cells in the injured brain. Acta Neurol Scand Suppl 67, 57:245.

Privat A (1975) Postnatal gliogenesis in the mammalian brain. Int Rev Cytol 40:281.

Roessman U, Friede RL (1968). Entry of labeled monocytic cells into the central nervous system. Acta Neuropath (Berlin) 10:359.

Russell GV (1962). The compound granular corpuscle or gitter cell: A review, together with notes on the origin of this phagocyte. Tex Rep Biol Med 20:338.

Schelper RL, Adrian EK (in press). Non-specific esterase activity in reactive cells in injured nervous tissue labeled with ^{3}H-thymidine or [125]Iododeoxyuridine injected before injury. J Comp Neur.

Schmalzl F, Braunsteiner H (1970). The cytochemistry of monocytes and macrophages. Ser Haemat 3:93.

Shnitka, TK, Seligman, AM (1961). Role of esteratic inhibition on localization of esterase and the simultaneous cytochemical demonstration of inhibitor sensitive and resistant enzyme species. J Histochem Cytochem 9:505.

Sjöstrand J (1971). Neuroglial proliferation in the hypoglossal nucleus after nerve injury. Exp Neurol 30:178.

Smith CW, Walker BE (1967). Glial and lymphoid cell response to tumor implantation in mouse brain. Tex Rep Biol Med 25:585.

Stenwig, AE (1972). The origin of brain macrophages in traumatic lesions, Wallerian degeneration, and retrograde degeneration. J Neuropath Exp Neurol 31:696.

Vaughn JE, Hinds PH, Skoff RP (1970). Electron microscopic studies of Wallerian degeneration in rat optic nerves. I. The multipotential glia. J Comp Neur 140:175.

Vaughn JE, Peters A (1968). A third neuroglial cell type. An electron microscope study. J Comp Neur 133:269.

Vaughn JE, Skoff RP (1972). Neuroglia in experimentally altered central nervous system. In Bourne, GH (ed): "The Structure and Function of Nervous Tissue," New York: Academic Press, p. 39.

Walker BE (1963). Infiltration and transformation of lymphoid cells in areas of spinal cord injury. Tex Rep Biol Med 21:615.

Williams RP, Adrian EK (1978). Prolonged availability of ^{3}H-thymidine following parenteral administration. Anat Rec 190:583.

Williams RP, Adrian EK (1980). Tritiated thymidine: systemic reutilization in the mouse. Anat Rec 196:206A.

Young MB (1977a). Effect of bilateral nerve injury on the migration of labelled mononuclear cells to hypoglossal nuclei. J Neuropath Exp Neurol 36:74.

Young MB (1977b). [3]HT-labelled blood cells in the CNS response to axotomies at various times after isotope injection. J Neuropath Exp Neurol 36:465.

Eleventh International Congress of Anatomy:
Glial and Neuronal Cell Biology, pages 125 – 139
© 1981 Alan R. Liss, Inc., 150 Fifth Avenue, New York, NY 10011

ORIGIN OF MICROGLIA: CELL TRANSFORMATION FROM BLOOD MONO-
CYTES INTO MACROPHAGIC AMEBOID CELLS AND MICROGLIA

Kikuko Imamoto

Department of Anatomy
Shiga University of Medical Science
Ohtsu, Shiga 520-21 Japan

INTRODUCTION

A concept of microglia was first proposed by del Rio-
Hortega during the years from 1919 to 1921, when the author
described their normal morphology, transformation to phagocytic cells, histogenesis and general distribution in the
central nervous system (Rio-Hortega, 1932). Later, there
was some confusion in the description of microglia and oligodendroglia on the basis of Hortega's silver carbonate
method. At present, however, with the introduction of
electron microscopy it is generally accepted that microglia
are a distinct type of glia with specific ultrastructural
features and phagocytic activity in the normal adult brain
(Mori and Leblond, 1969).

The origin of microglia is still a matter of controversy.
Some investigators consider that microglia are probably derived from the neuroectoderm as are other macroglia (Lewis,
1968; Vaughn and Skoff, 1972; Fujita and Kitamura, 1975);
others follow the view of del Rio-Hortega in proposing that
microglia come from mesenchymal elements (Cammermeyer, 1970;
Stensaas, 1975). Moreover, the relationship between microglia and brain macrophages remains to be resolved. Although
it is widely known that active phagocytes increase in
number in the wound area it is not known whether the precursors of such active phagocytes are intrinsic cells or extrinsic. The phagocytic function of resting microglia may
be activated in the damaged brain (Cammermeyer, 1970; Penfield, 1932), but there are many reports suggesting that
active phagocytes are macrophages derived from blood mononuclear cells, probably monocytes (Koningsmark and Sidman,

1963; Stenwig, 1972; Kitamura et al., 1972).

In the present paper, we summarize a series of experiments on the origin of microglia, performed with the hope of finding relationships among monocytes, macrophages in the wounded brain and ameboid cells in the neonatal brain. Most of these experiments have been done in collaboration with Dr. C.P. Leblond at McGill University in Montreal, Canada.

MATERIAL AND METHOD

1) In order to examine the possibility of transformation from hematogenous cells to macrophages, we have done the following experiments (Imamoto and Leblond, 1977).

Bone marrow cells of inbred Lewis rats were isolated and incubated for 1 hour in medium containing ^{3}H-uridine. After washing out free radioactive uridine, all the labeled marrow cells was intravenously injected into recipient rats given a stab wound in the cerebral cortex either 30 min before or after cell injection. Rats were sacrificed at various times and Epon serial sections were prepared for radioautography.

2) In order to examine the formation of microglia in the corpus callosum, we injected ^{3}H-thymidine into rats in four groups, that is, 100g (30 day old), 80g (25 day old), 40g (19 day old) and 15 g (5 day old) rats. Rats given 3 i.p. injections (4 μCi/gbw: at 7 hour intervals) were sacrificed from 1 to 28 days after injection. Rats given a single injection (20 μCi/gbw) were sacrificed at 2 hours. Then, Epon serial sections were prepared for radioautography (Imamoto et al., 1978).

3) In order to follow the cell transformation from ameboid cells to microglia, a fluorescent dye, primulin, was intravenously injected into newborn rats (12 μl of 10% primulin dissolved in saline). Rats were perfused by Faglu solution and brains were immersed overnight in Faglu sucrose solution. Cryostat sections of 14 μ in thickness were examined under an incident fluorescence microscope.

RESULTS AND DISCUSSION

Microglia are characterized by a small nucleus with dense clumps of chromatin and a scanty cytoplasm often extending into ramified processes, in which there are lysosomal dense bodies, a few long strands of rough endoplasmic reticulum and occasionally the Golgi apparatus (Fig. 1). These features are common in so-called resting microglia reported in various animals (Vaughn and Peters, 1971; Stensaas and Stensaas, 1968; Mori and Leblond, 1969; Phillips, 1973).

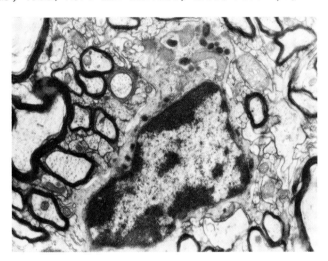

Figure 1. Microglia in the corpus callosum. x14,000.

Even under a light microscope, microglia are identified quite easily in semithin sections stained with toluidine blue, because their nuclei are more deeply stained than those of oligodendrocytes and astrocytes (Fig. 9). This technique for the identification of glia cells has been regarded as reliable enough to correspond with the data obtained by electron microscopy and used in our work (Ling et al., 1973).

ORIGIN OF MACROPHAGES IN THE STAB WOUND

Ultrastructure of Macrophages

In the wound area, considerable cell accumulation was noted within the first few days. Among the hematogenous

cells, macrophages were easily identified because of the presence of numerous phagosomes in the cytoplasm. Remnants of
red blood cells and irregular residual bodies were often seen
in the main part of the cytoplasm, in addition to lipid droplets and primary or secondary lysosomes. In addition, an
ovoid or kidney-shaped nucleus located eccentrically, an extensive Golgi field, long cisterns of rough endoplasmic reticulum, vacuoles with fluffy materials and filopodia on the
cell surface were characteristic of brain macrophages (Fig.
2). Some of these features seemed to belong to blood monocytes. Actually, in the open wound there were a number of
cells showing intermediate forms between macrophages and monocytes, suggesting a close relationship between these cell
types.

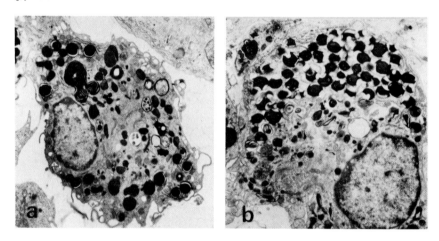

Figure 2. Two typical macrophages with various types of
phagosomes in the wound area. A: x4,500, B: x5,000.

Radioautography of Transfused Bone Marrow Cells

Our first experiment required dozens of radioautographic
slides to find labeled cells in the wound area. After a
careful survey of many slides, a total of only 220 cells
was recorded on the wound side of 18 experimental rats,
whereas no labeled cells were found on the control side.
(Table 1.)

The transfused marrow cell appeared as brain macrophages
(over 100 cells) in the open wound in the first 3 days
(Fig. 3). In addition, 39 granulocytes, 48 monocytes and

Time after wound (days)	Number of rats with		Number of labeled cells					
	Total	labeled cells	Granulo-cytes	Mono-cytes	Macro-phages	Micro-glia	Uniden-tified	Total
1d	5	4	22	18	7	7	9	63
2	8	6	5	15	24	1	1	46
3	4	4	12	14	61	3	3	93
5	1	1	0	1	6	0	0	7
6	1	1	0	0	3	0	0	3
7	3	1	0	0	6	1	0	7
8	1	1	0	0	0	0	1	1
10-15	6	0	0	0	0	0	0	0
	29	18	39	48	107	12	14	220

Table 1. Labeled cells appeared in the region of the wound.

12 microglia were identified during the 8 days after wounding. Thereafter, no labeled cells were found, probably because of the turnover of radioactive uridine incorporated into cytoplasmic RNA. Labeled marrow cells regarded as microglia were small cells with a dark nucleus enclosed by a thin basophilic cytoplasm (Fig. 4). Most labeled microglia were observed either in a satellite position by a neuron or in the perivascular area adjacent to the wound. Two labeled microglia were present in the subependymal layer quite far from the wound at 1 and 3 days after wounding. In these regions, microglia tend to predominate even under normal conditions (Cammermeyer, 1970). Hence, we considered that the transfused marrow cells, probably monocytes, could give rise directly to microglia and macrophages.

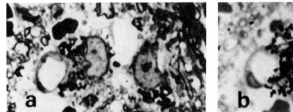 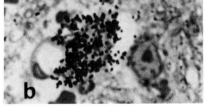

Figure 3. Macrophage in the stab wound (a). Radioautograph shows many silver grains over the cell (b). x1,500.

Since the labels disappeared after 8 days, we could not follow the fate of labeled macrophages for a long time.

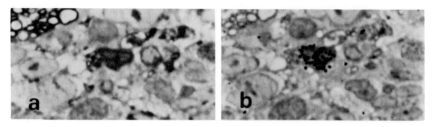

Figure 4. Microglia in the subependyma 1 day after wounding (a). This cell is covered with silver grains (b). x1,500.

However, it was noted that the size of macrophages tended to diminish with time, and thus microglia-like cells with a small dark nucleus and a few phagosomes gradually increased in number in the healing part of the wound. These microglia-like cells were not related to the endogenous microglia, since mobility and mitotic activity were hardly seen in the endogenous microglia around the wound before the appearance of microglia-like cells. Later, however, astrocytic proliferation was observed in the healing part.

The percentages of the most numerous cell types, after counting a total of 300 cells in the wound area of each animal, are reported in Fig. 5. The graphs of macrophages and microglia-like cells indicate a sequential transformation from the former to the latter.

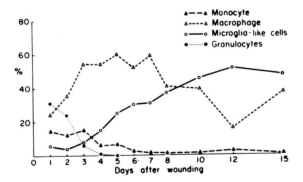

Figure 5. Graph showing the average percentage of the various cell types in the wound.

Our first experiment provided direct evidence that blood monocytes give rise to macrophages and evidence that macrophages evolve into microglia-like cells, which may become microglia in turn. Some microglia, however, seem to come from blood monocytes by a direct transformation. In either case monocytes would be the initial precursors of microglia.

RELATIONSHIP BETWEEN AMEBOID CELLS AND MICROGLIA IN THE NEONATAL BRAIN

Mitosis of Microglia

An entirely different approach to the formation of microglia was tried in a series of experiments following i.p. injections of ^{3}H-thymidine into 100g, 80g and 40g rats (Mori and Leblond, 1969; Imamoto et al., 1978).

Although active gliogenesis was confirmed in the rapidly growing rats, no labeled microglia were seen 2 hours after ^{3}H-thymidine injection. Furthermore, labeled microglia were rarely observed even at the later time. From these data we considered that microglia had no ability to divide under normal conditions and that the bulk of them must be formed at an early stage of life. Hence, we continued to search for the formation of microglia in 5 day old rats, in which the corpus callosum was composed of immature cells or glioblasts and another cell type called ameboid cells.

Ultrastructure of Ameboid Cells

An ameboid cell has a large ovoid nucleus with a prominent nucleolus and a spongy cytoplasm showing an irregular surface with invaginations and filopodia (Fig. 6). Lysosomal dense bodies and vacuoles with fluffy materials often spread throughout the cytoplasm, and occasionally pleomorphic residual bodies and lipid droplets are also seen. These overall features of ameboid cells closely resemble those of macrophages observed in wounds. Some of the ameboid cells are very similar to the monocytes. Ameboid cells usually predominate in the area with loose structure in the brain parenchyma only in the early postnatal period.

The presence of ameboid cells in the neonatal stage has already been reported in rabbit (Stensaas and Reichert, 1971; Ferrer and Serimento, 1980), chicken (Booz and Felsing, 1973),

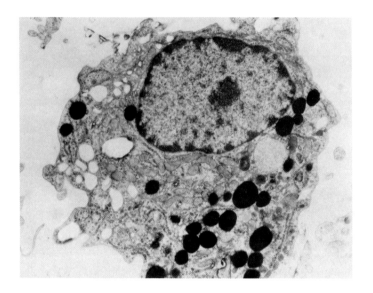

Figure 6.   Electron micrograph of an ameboid cell.   x9,200.

mice (Fujita and Kitamura, 1976) and rats (Caley and Maxwell, 1968; Ling and Tan, 1976). However, the origin of ameboid cells and their fate have not been determined yet.

Number of Ameboid Cells

Ameboid cells constituted 7% of the cell population in the corpus callosum in 5 day old rats (Table 2). As time elapsed the callosal fibers became packed and myelinated, accompanying the differentiation of oligodendrocytes and astrocytes. At the age of 12 days, typical microglia were present in substantial numbers, and by 19 days the number doubled to reach a plateau with about 2%, while ameboid cells had completely disappeared from the corpus callosum.

We found many intermediate cells between ameboid cells and microglia and also degenerating ameboid cells, and esti- mated that about one third of the ameboid cells would trans- form into microglia, while the rest would die. A possible sequence of cell transformation of ameboid cells was pro- posed as shown in Fig. 7.

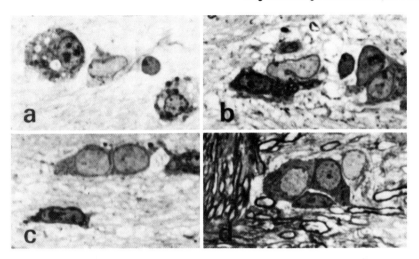

Figure 7. A sequence of cell transformation from ameboid cell to typical microglia in the corpus callosum. x1,500.
a: Two typical ameboid cells in a 5d-old rat.
b: Transforming ameboid cell in a 9d-old rat.
c: Microglia-like cell in a 12d-old rat.
d: Typical microglia in a 19d-old rat.

Age of rat	Number of rats	Immature cells (glioblast)	Ameboid cells	Micro-glia	Total glia counted
5d	4	44.7 ᵇ	7.2 ᵇ	0.3 ᵇ	673
6	4	42.6	6.6	0.4	792
7	4	38.9	5.1	0.3	724
9	3	35.7	8.8	0.6	724
12	4	38.2	2.4	1.2	727
19	3	22.5	0.0	2.1	913
26	3	19.5	0.0	2.7	918
33	3	15.5	0.0	2.1	898

The numbers are expressed as average percent.

Table 2. Glial index in 14 g rat series.

Labeling Index in 15 g Rat Series

Although microglia themselves were not capable of mitosis under normal conditions, new microglia appearing with time were labeled prominently. Presumably, such micro-glia must have come from the other cell type which had been initially labeled with ^{3}H-thymidine (Fig. 8).

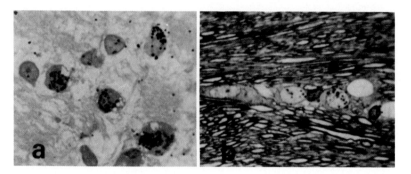

Figure 8. Radioautographs of the corpus callosum.
a: Three labeled ameboid cells intermingling with immature cells, of which one is labeled 2 d after injection.
b: Two labeled microglia seen in a row of glia cells 28 d after ^{3}H-thymidine injection. x1,000.

Immature cells or glioblasts and ameboid cells were labeled at 2 hours after ^{3}H-thymidine injection. Therefore, both had the possibility to become the precursors of the labeled microglia.

As shown in Fig. 9, the labeling index of immature cells reached a peak of 60% at 4 days after injection (9 day old) and declined slowly, while that of ameboid cells showed a peak of 78% at 7 days (12 day old). At that time microglia appeared with a high labeling index. As a matter of fact, the total number of microglia was rather small in 12 day old rats, but we noted their labeling index of 80%. Comparing the labeling index of immature cells with that of ameboid cells, the height of the peak pointed to the latter as precursors of the highly labeled microglia. Though ameboid cells were no longer seen at 14 days after injection, the high labeling index of microglia always exceeded any other indices, which generally dropped down after reaching their peaks, up to 28 days after injection. For example, the labeling indices of immature cells, oligodendrocytes and astrocytes were about 16%, 56% and 20% respectively at 28 days after injection (unpublished data).

These data indicated that the labeling index of microglia was quite different from those of oligodendrocytes and astrocytes derived from glioblasts. Microglia appearing in the corpus callosum probably resulted from the transformation of the ameboid cells during the first 3 weeks of life.

The conclusion in the 15 g rat series was that ameboid cells in the neonatal rats might be fated to become typical microglia with the maturation of brain structure (Imamoto and Leblond, 1978).

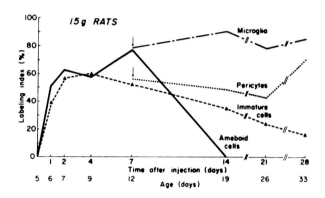

Figure 9.   Labeling index in 15 g rat series.

Transformation of Ameboid Cells to Microglia

A successive transformation from ameboid cells to typical microglia was seen in Epon semithin sections stained with toluidine blue (Fig. 7). Thus, we confirmed this event in the neonatal rats receiving the fluorescent dye, primulin.

In normal newborn rats, a small number of spherical cells with weak yellow fluorescence were seen in the subarachnoid space and in the corpus callosum. The spherical cells in the subarachnoid space were regarded as mast cells with fluorescence of amines, whereas those in the corpus callosum were probably ameboid cells containing lipofuscin-like dense materials with autofluorescence.

At 3 days after primulin injection, spherical cells with strong fluorescence accumulated on the surface of the brain and in the corpus callosum. They were probably blood monocytes in the pia mater and ameboid cells in the corpus callosum, becoming macrophagic cells. Phagocytized primulin showed strong fluorescence within the cytoplasm (Fig. 10). With time ameboid cells with primulin became elongated. Instead of spherical ameboid cells, ramified microglia-like cells became scattered throughout the corpus callosum, showing strong yellow fluorescence, at 14 days after primulin injection (Fig. 11). It is almost coincident with the time of appearance of typical microglia. These observations support our view on the transformation of ameboid cells to microglia.

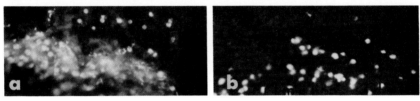

Figure 10. Spherical cells showing fluorescence of primulin 3 days after injection. Numerous monocytes migrate into the pia mater and some into the subarachnoid space, located in the upper right (a). Ameboid cells in the corpus callosum also show strong fluorescence (b).   x250.

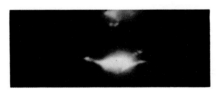

Figure 11. Microglia in the corpus callosum 14 days after injection of primulin. Note the ramified processes.   x1,500.

Origin of Ameboid Cells

Finally, it should be confirmed by a direct method whether or not blood monocytes give rise to ameboid cells in the early postnatal period. In order to solve this problem, Ling et al. (1980) recently carried out the following experiment.

Inbred adult rats received intravenous injections of carbon particles. Twenty-four hours after, carbon labeled monocytes were separated from the circulating blood in Percoll gradient solution. Then a suspension containing 80% monocytes and 20% lymphocytes was transfused into newborn rats.

Five days after injection of labeled monocytes carbon labeled ameboid cells appeared in the corpus callosum. Even though the labeled ameboid cells in the corpus callosum were few in number, it was unquestionable that the transfused monocytes turned into ameboid cells in the corpus callosum of 5 day old rats.

This direct evidence strongly supports our speculation on the monocytal origin of ameboid cells.

CONCLUSION

Our conclusion on the origin of microglia is summarized in Fig. 12.

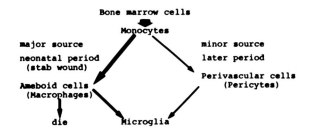

Figure 12. Origin of microglia.

Blood monocytes enter the brain parenchyma in the early postnatal period, and settle as monocytic ameboid cells which evolve into somewhat macrophagic ameboid cells. Between the second and the third weeks, macrophagic ameboid cells disappear from the corpus callosum, probably because some of them die and the rest, about one third, become typical microglia. This is the major source of microglia under normal conditions.

Similarly, in the case of the stab wound monocytes enter the brain through the open wound and become macrophages, some of which may die; the rest remain as microglia in the healing part of the wound.

As a minor source of microglia at a later period, we saw that new cells rarely arise through the stage of perivascular cells or pericytes.

Therefore, monocytes would be the initial precursors of microglia both in the neonatal period and in adult life.

ACKNOWLEDGEMENT
The author is grateful to Dr. T. Maeda and Dr. S. Fedoroff for kindly reading this manuscript.

REFERENCES

Booz KH, Felsing T (1973). Uber ein transitorisches perinatales subependymales Zellsystem der weissen Ratte. Z Anat Entwicklungsgesch 141:275.

Caley DN, Maxwell DS (1968). An electron microscopic study of the neuroglia during postnatal development of the rat cerebrum. J Comp Neur 133:45.

Cammermeyer J (1970). The life history of the microglia cell: A light microscopic study. Neuroscience Res 3:43.

Ferrer I, Sarmiento J (1980). Nascent microglia in the developing brain. Acta Neuropathol (Berl) 50:61.

Fujita S, Kitamura T (1975). Origin of brain macrophages and the nature of the so-called microglia. Acta Neuropathol (Berl) Suppl VI:291.

Fujita S, Kitamura T (1976). Origin of brain macrophages and the nature of the microglia. In Zimmermann HM (ed) Progress in neuropathology vol III Grune and Stratton, London p. 1.

Imamoto K, Leblond CP (1977). Presence of labeled monocytes, macrophages and microglia in a stab wound of the brain following an injection of bone marrow cells labeled with ^{3}H-thymidine into rats. J Comp Neur 174:255.

Imamoto K, Leblond CP (1978). Radioautographic investigation of gliogenesis in the corpus callosum of young rats. II. Origin of microglial cells. J Comp Neur 180:139.

Imamoto K, Paterson JA, Leblond CP (1978). Radioautographic investigation of gliogenesis in the corpus callosum of young rats. I. Sequential changes in oligodendrocytes. J Comp Neur 180:115.

Kitamura T, Hattori H, Fujita S (1972). Autoradiographic studies on histogenesis of brain macrophages in the mouse. J Neuropathol exp Neur 31:502.

Konigsmark BW, Sidman RL (1963). Origin of brain macrophages in the mouse. J Neuropathol exp Neur 22:643.

Lewis PD (1968). The fate of the subependymal cell in the adult rat brain with a note on the origin of microglia. Brain 91:721.

Ling EA, Paterson AJ, Privat A, Mori S, Leblond CP (1973). Investigation of glial cells in the semithin sections. I. Identification of glial cells in the brain of young rats. J Comp Neur 149:43.

Ling EA, Penny D, Leblond CP (1980). Use of carbon labeling to demonstrate the role of blood monocytes as precursors of the "ameboid cells" present in the corpus callosum of postnatal rat. J Comp Neur in press.

Ling EA and Tan CK (1974). Ameboid microglial cells in the corpus callosum of neonatal rats. Archiv histol Jap 36: 265.

Mori S, Leblond CP (1969). Identification of microglia in light and electron microscopy. J Comp Neur 135:57.

Penfield W (1932). Neuroglia. In Penfield W (ed) Cytology and cellular pathology of the nervous system. Paul B Hoeber Inc New York.

Phillips DE (1973). An electron microscopic study of macroglia and microglia in the lateral funiculus of the developing spinal cord in the fetal monkey. Z Zellforsch 140:145.

del Rio-Hortega P (1932). Microglia. In Penfield W (ed) Cytology and cellular pathology of the nervous system. Paul B Hoeber Inc New York vol II p. 483.

Stensaas LJ (1975). Pericytes and perivascular microglia cells in the basal forebrain of neonatal rabbit. Cell Tiss Res 158:517.

Stensass LJ, Reichert WH (1971). Round and ameboid microglial cells in the neonatal rabbit brain. Z Zellforsch 119:147.

Stensaas LJ, Stensaas S (1968). Astrocytic neuroglial cells, oligodendrocytes and microgliacytes in the spinal cord of the toad. Z Zellforsch 86:184.

Stenwig AE (1972). The origin of brain macrophages in traumatic lesions, Wallerian degeneration and retrograde degeneration. J Neuropathol exp Neur 31:695.

Vaughn DW, Peters A (1971). The morphology and development of neuroglial cells. In Pease DC (ed) Cellular aspects of neural growth and differentiation. Univ. of California Press, Berkeley p. 103.

Vaughn JE, Skoff RP (1972). Neuroglia in experimentally altered central nervous system. In Bourne GH (ed) The structure and function of nervous tissue. New York: Acad Press, p. 39.

Eleventh International Congress of Anatomy:
Glial and Neuronal Cell Biology, pages 141—169
© **1981 Alan R. Liss, Inc., 150 Fifth Avenue, New York, NY 10011**

ORIGIN, MORPHOLOGY AND FUNCTION OF THE MICROGLIA

S.Fujita, Y.Tsuchihashi and T.Kitamura

Department of Pathology,
Kyoto Prefectural University of Medicine
Kawaramachi, Kyoto 602, Japan

INTRODUCTION:
A CRITICAL SURVEY OF MICROGLIAL STUDY UP TO 1976

Sixty years ago, Del Rio-Hortega (1919,1921) suggested that the microglial cells are of embryonic polyblast origin migrating from the meninges and perivascular connective tissue in the last periods of embryonic life, and that they change into macrophages when the brain is damaged. Hortega's microglial theory has been universally accepted.

However, with introduction of ^{3}H-TdR ARG (tritiated thymidine autoradiography) and EM (electron microscopy), strong evidence has been accumulated to indicate that the source of supply of brain macrophages throughout life is to be found in circulating blood monocytes (Fujita and Kitamura 1976). The most significant evidence is the following.

(1) ARG experiments to follow the fate of leucocytes label- ed with ^{3}H-TdR have revealed that almost all the inflammatory cells and the brain macrophages are derived from circulating blood monocytes (cf. Fig. 1), irrespective of the type of neural damage: stab wound, viral encephalitis, and retrograde degeneration (Fujita and Kitamura 1975). It was generally believed among neuropathologists that the participation of hematogenous cells in viral encephalitis is restricted only to the perivascular cuffs, but the ARG experiments proved that all the inflammatory cells in acute stage of experimental Japanese encephalitis, including rod-shaped cells, cells forming glial nodules as well as those in perivascular cuffs,

are derived from circulating blood mononuclear leucocytes (Sato 1968, Kitamura et al. 1973).

(2) Comparison of labeling percentages of circulating blood monocytes and macrophages has led to a conclusion that the cells normally present in the adult brain do not participate in macrophage formation. Pericytes and the "resting" microglia therefore, are not precursors of the macrophages (Kitamura et al. 1972) (cf. Fig. 1).

(3) Electron microscopic investigation has demonstrated, in damaged brains, leucocytes being in the process of extravasation (Lampert 1967, Field and Raine 1969, Prineas et al. 1969, Baringer and Griffith 1970). These leucocytes temporarily take pericytal and adventitial positions. They are, however, not proper pericytes or adventitial cells. It was pointed out (Fujita and Kitamura 1976) that they are not found in the normal adult brain. In fact, they could be differentiated from the proper pericytes by their possession of the ^{3}H-label that served as a marker of leucocytes (Kitamura et al. 1972). Similar observations, but without the label seem to have led previous investigators to an erroneous conclusion that the "pericytes" or "adventitial cells" were the origin of the brain macrophages.

(4) Hortega's silver carbonate method rather selectively stains immature forms of neuroglial cells, particularly glioblasts when applied to the developing CNS. We have repeatedly pointed out this fact (Fujita 1966). However, it has not been widely known that Penfield, an intimate collaborator of Del Rio-Hortega, also utilized this method to stain glioblasts, which he called "new-formed spongioblasts" in "medullary canal of mouse of 9 days" (cf. Fig. 14 and p.444 of his article, 1932). This fact that the same silver carbonate method stains glioblasts in the developing CNS as well as the microglial cells and macrophages in the adult brain seems to have been a source of confusion of interrelationships between these three groups of cells. To avoid the confusion, we have proposed that the name of the microglia should be applied only to the so-called resting microglia that are present in the normal adult brain but never to the brain macrophages. The brain macrophages should be called as such. If we admit peculiar naming of "microglia" for the monocytes that infiltrate brain tissue, we should create as many names of leucocytes as numbers of organs exist in which inflammatory processes take place. To avoid such a nonsense, we have to

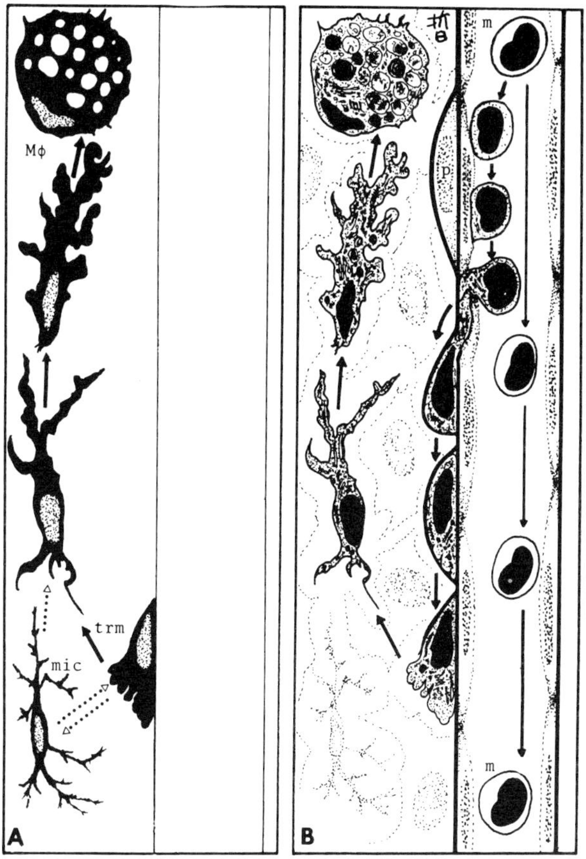

Fig. 1 When damaged brain tissue is examined by Hortega's silver carbonate method, a series of cells from transformed monocytes (trm) to macrophages (Mφ) together with the resting microglia (mic) are stained, but monocytes in the blood stream or in the process of extravasation are not impregnated as shown in Schema A. Inevitably, the resting microglia (mic) were taken for the source of the macrophage. However, if the same material is examined by EM-ARG after selective labeling of nuclear DNA, as indicated with black nuclei, of circulating leucocytes, it becomes evident that true precursors of the macrophages are circulating monocytes (m), as shown in Schema B. The pericytes (p) and the microglia do not contribute to the macrophage formation. (For evidences that support this schema, cf. Fujita and Kitamura 1976)

reject the customary usage of "microglia" to designate brain macrophages. In the present paper, we adhere strictly to this rule. Only the cells that have been called the "resting microglia" and those that are proved to have directly changed from them are called microglia.

(5) Monocytes once infiltrated the nervous tissue are capable of temporary proliferation and may increase in number (Hattori 1973). But they cannot be permanent residents in the normal CNS. When the damage to the nervous tissue has subsided to a normal condition, they disappear either by disintegration or/and by re-entrance into the vascular lumina (Fujita and Kitamura 1976). These findings make the hypothesis unlikely that the hematogenous elements may infiltrate the CNS at embryonic stages to persist into adult life as a permanent source of the brain macrophages.

(6) In our previous studies on cytogenesis of the CNS, it was demonstrated that the microglia are differentiated together with other neuroglial cells at a later stage of prenatal development. In the earliest stage of development of the CNS the neural tube is composed solely of matrix cells. Neither neuroblasts (syn. immature neurons) nor spongioblasts (hypothetical precursors of neuroglia, His 1889) are produced. We call this stage as stage I of cytogenesis of the CNS (Fujita 1963). However, soon this stage of pure matrix cell proliferation ends and neuroblasts begin to be produced from matrix cells. This is stage II of cytogenesis or stage of neuron production (Fujita 1964). Glial cell lines are not yet differentiated at this stage (Fujita 1963, 1964, 1966, Fujita and Kitamura 1976). Therefore, matrix cells forming a radial frame work of the neural tube play a role of supportive elements which Ramon y Cajal called "cellule épitheliale primitive" (1908). When the neuroblast production comes to an end, stage III begins (Fujita 1963, 1964). Now remaining matrix cells change into ependymoglioblasts (epgb in Fig. 2) which, though having lost their potential to produce neurons, can be hardly differentiated morphologically from matrix cells. The ependymoglioblasts are transitional intermediate forms and change rapidly into ependymal cells and glioblasts (Fujita 1963, Fujita and Fujita 1964, Fujita 1964, 1965, 1973). When the glioblasts are produced at stage III of cytogenesis some are accumulated in the subependymal layer, many migrate into deep parenchyma and others reach subpial or marginal layers. They differentiate, as development proceeds, astroglia, oligodendroglia and microglia, sequentially (Fig. 2).

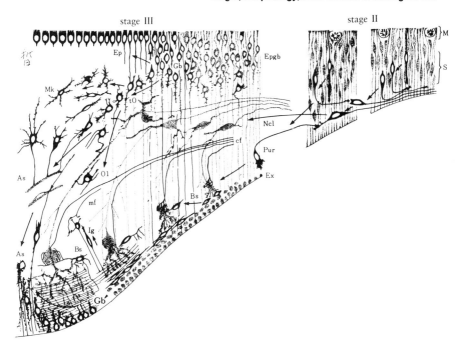

Fig. 2 Schematic representation of cytogenesis in the
brain and cerebellum at stage II and stage III of cytogenesis.
M indicate M-zone and S, S-zone of matrix layer. Epgb means
ependymoglioblast; Gb, glioblasts; Gb', glioblasts in the
external granular layer of the cerebellum; Ep, ependymal
cells; tO, transitory oligodendroglia; Mk, microglia; O1,
oligodendroglia; As, astroglia. Ncl indicates neurons of
cerebellar nuclei; Pur, Purkinje cells; Ex, external matrix
layer; cf, climbing fiber; Bs, basket neurons; mf, mossy
fiber; Ig, internal granular neurons. (Modified from
Fujita and Kitamura 1976).

So we came to a conclusion that the resting microglia are
the third subspecies of neuroglia, unrelated to the reticulo-
endothelial system (Fujita and Kitamura 1976). This was the
status praesens of our knowledge on the microglia in 1976.

There is a traditional belief, however, that the microglia themselves are monocytes that have infiltrated the nervous tissue at a late stage of embryonic development. Evidence
for this belief, as far as we have investigated from the

literature, is practically lacking. And Del Rio-Hortega
(1932) as well as Ramon y Cajal excluded this possibility
since the microglia and blood monocytes stain so differently
by the silver carbonate method; circulating blood monocytes
are not stained at all. Ramon y Cajal pointed out that:
"Por otra parte, los leucocitos intravasculares observados
en las preparaciones donde la microglia se tiñe intensa y
completamente no atraen ni poco ni mucho la plata coloidal"
(1920). Nevertheless, this traditional belief prevails widely among modern investigators. Therefore, it is necessary to
examine critically this hypothesis by modern techniques. We
have attacked this problem from two different apporaches;
Immunohistochemical comparison of the microglia with blood
monocytes and macrophages (Tsuchihashi et al. 1977, Fujita et
al. 1978), and ultrastructural study on the microglia in
normal and pathologic conditions (Kitamura et al. 1977, 1978).
Both lines of the research were, at the same time, planned
to examine refutability of those conclusions (1) through (6)
mentioned above.

ORIGIN OF THE MICROGLIA AS EXAMINED BY IMMUNOHISTOCHEMISTRY

        In order to examine whether the microglia in the normal
brain have any relationship to monocytes, we prepared anti-
leucocyte antibody and examined its reaction with the microglia, monocytes, macrophages and other kinds of cells by immunohistochemical technique. The antibody was produced in rabbits
by injecting whole cell suspension of monocyte-macrophage
mixture collected from rat peritoneal exudates. Peritoneal
exudates were obtained from Donryu rats 4 days after intraperitoneal injection of 5 ml of 5% glucose solution in which
3% of liquid paraffin was suspended. In earlier experiments,
we tried to purify the antigen by various techniques as described by Unanue (1968) and others but soon we learnt that
the merely washed suspension of the monocyte-macrophage rich
peritoneal exudate gave more satisfactory results if absorp-
tion of the antiserum was performed with rat ascites hepatoma
cells AH13. The antiserum taken from the rabbit was heat in-
activated and absorbed by the AH13 cells for 2 hrs. This
procedure is much better than that with liver powder to raise
specificity of the antiserum, probably because the former
contains small amount of lymphocytes, mast cells, constituent
of ascitic fluid, etc. besides AH13 hepatoma cells. To stain
sections of brain, spleen, thymus, and so on and smears of
peripheral blood and ascites, standard technique of indirect

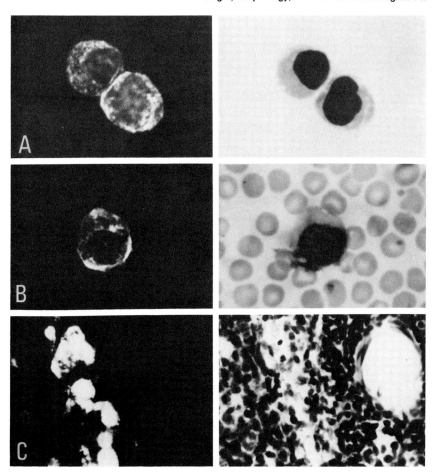

Fig. 3 A: Peritoneal monocyte-macrophages reacted strongly
with this antiserum. B: Monocytes in the peripheral blood
also showed brilliant fluorescence. C: Section of thymus.
Only macrophages were reactive. Endothelial cells, fibroblasts, lymphocytes were totally non-reactive.

immunofluorescence staining was performed. After fluorescence
observation of the antigen-antibody reaction, the specimen was
washed and stained by hematoxylin eosin or by Giemsa. The same
cells were identified and studied under a light microscope.
<u>Results</u>
In the peritoneal fluid, macrophages, monocytes and neutrophil
leucocytes were reactive (Fig. 3) with the antiserum.

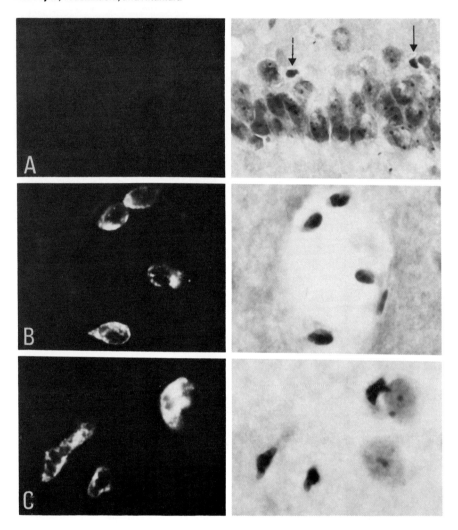

Fig. 4 Sections of brain. A: Normal rat hippocampus, pyramidal cell layer. Nuclei indicated by arrows are those of
microglial cells. The microglia do not react with the anti-
leucocyte antiserum. Neurons, neuroglia, pericytes, endothelial cells are also totally non-reactive. B: After stab
wounding, many monocytes are attached to blood vessel wall
and begin to extravasate. C: 4 days after stab wounding.
Now many cells strongly reactive with the antiserum appear
in the brain parenchyma. Judged from their morphology and
distribution, they are transformed monocytes and macrophages.

Monocytes in the peripheral blood also reacted positively
(Fig. 3B). In sections of spleen and thymus (Fig. 3C), all
the lymphocytes, reticulum cells, endothelial cells, fibroblasts, smooth muscle cells failed to show the fluorescence.
Only macrophages reacted positively (Fig. 3C). It was clear
that the antiserum reacts only with macrophages, monocytes,
and granulocytes, but not with T- and B-lymphocytes.

Normal brain tissue was examined. No cells in the brain parenchyma showed positive fluorescence. None of the pericytes
and other perivascular cells reacted positively. It was evident that the microglia are totally non-reactive (Fig. 4A).
Sections of cerebral hemispheres including hippocampus, subependymal layers, corpus callosum and diencephalon were tested but only free leucocytes in the vascular lumen and a few
cells in pia-arachnoidal tissue reacted positively.

Injured brain tissue
After stab wounds, blood vessels in the brain parenchyma
frequently showed monocytes attached to the vascular wall or
in the process of extravasation (Fig. 4B). They reacted
strongly with the antiserum. In the brain parenchyma, there
were many cells that reacted with the anti-leucocyte antiserum (Fig. 4C). Their distribution, shape and nuclear and
cytoplasmic morphology indicated that they are the inflammatory cells and macrophages that had been identified as transformed monocytes by ^{3}H-TdR ARG in earlier studies.
Very frequently perineuronal satellites (Fig. 4C) showed
brilliant fluorescence thereby indicating their monocytic
origin.

From these observations we concluded (Tsuchihashi et al.
1977, Fujita et al. 1978) that:
(1) Brain macrophages and their precursors in the brain are
derived from circulating blood monocytes at the time of
injuries,
(2) In normal rat brain parenchyma, hematogenous cells are
not present,
(3) Therefore, the resting microglia are definitively
different from hematogenous cells,
(4) The microglia cannot be of hematogenous origin.

Similar observations have been reported using anti-macrophage
and anti-S100 antibodies (Persson et al. 1978), anti-lympho-
cyte, anti-monocyte sera (Oehmichen et al. 1979) and macrophage sepecific anti-serum and IgG Fc receptor assay (Wood et
al. 1979). It is remarkable that all these authors, working
independently, reached a unanimous conclusion that the micro-

glia are not derived from mononuclear blood cells, and that all the inflammatory macrophages are derived from hematogenous precursors. These conclusions fit nicely into the histogenetic scheme of the microglia as presented in Fig. 5 (cf. Fujita and Kitamura 1976 for this scheme) that the microglia belong to and form the third subspecies of neuroglia while macrophages are exclusively derived from circulating blood monocytes.

MORPHOLOGY OF THE MICROGLIAL CELLS

Before we can discuss any morphological difference or similarity between the microglia and other kinds of cells such as blood cells, it is absolutely necessary to identify microglial cells under an electron microscope. This is not an easy task, as it may appear. Earlier we attempted to study electron microscopic morphology of typical resting microglia in the rabbit hippocampus where abundant silver carbonate-

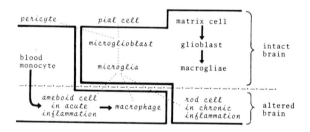

Fig. 5 Origin of brain macrophages and other inflammatory cells and the nature of the microglia. Classical concept of microglia system is shown in italics connected with dotted lines. In this scheme we propose that amoeboid inflammatory cells and macrophages are exclusively derived from circulating blood monocytes, irrespective of the types of neural damage. Indigenous cells in the adult normal brain, i.e. proper pericytes and the microglia, do not contribute to macrophage formation. The so-called resting microglia and the microglioblasts belong to neuroglia of matrix cell origin. The microglia constitute the third subspecies of neuroglia. As a consequence, the microglia system of Hortega is separated into two groups of cells different in origin and function as indicated by bold lines; monocyte-macrophage system and system of neuroglial cells.

positive cells must be present. We could not demonstrate
any dark cells that might be definitively different from
other glial cells nor were there cells that bore morphological characteristics of hematogenous cells. The problem was that
we did not have any means to decide which cell is the microglia. Mori and Leblond (1969) used silver carbonate staining to identify the microglia in EM. However, fixation of
their original method deteriorates fine-structure of the
nervous tissue drastically.

We modified the procedure using 3% formaldehyde perfusion
via ascending aorta followed by "isotonic bromification" so
that the specimen gives satisfactory detail of the fine-
structure of the nervous tissue if silver staining is omitted
(Kitamura et al. 1977). After the perfusion, hippocampal
area of the rabbit was cut out and post-fixed for 30 min in
"isotonic brom formalin" which was prepared by adding 0.4g
of ammonium bromide and 2 ml of neutral formalin to 20 ml of
5% glucose solution. Then the sections were stained with
silver carbonate for 30 sec to 2 min and reduced in 4% formaldehyde according to the original method of Del Rio-Hortega
(1919). For EM, the sections were treated in osmium tetroxide
solution, dehydrated and embedded in epoxy resin. For conventional EM, adjacent Vibratome sections were taken and processed as usual. First we confirmed, by light microscopy of
semithin sections, that the typical microglial cells were
selectively stained. Thin sections were cut out from the
same block and examined by an electron microscope. All the
cells stained with the silver carbonate appeared dark due to
deposit of the silver salt. Approximately 20% of non-neuronal
cells in the stratum radiatum of rabbit hippocampus were the
microglial cells. The cells stained selectively with the
silver carbonate showed some common features (Fig. 6B). Their
nuclear shape was variable but usually elongated. The nucleus
possessed clumped chromatin of which most was attached to
the nuclear membrane. Scanty cytoplasm in the perikaryon continued to thin cytoplasmic processes. In general, preservation
of the fine-structure after the silver impregnation was poor
but we could recognize morphological characteristics that
may serve as markers to identify the microglia in conventional electron micrographs (Fig. 6B): configuration and contour
of the cell, shape of the nucleus, pattern of chromatin distribution, scanty cytoplasm in the perikaryon that contains
characteristic organelles, branching of spine-like processes
and so on. Examination of conventional electron micrographs
taken from the adjacent Vibratome section revealed the occur-

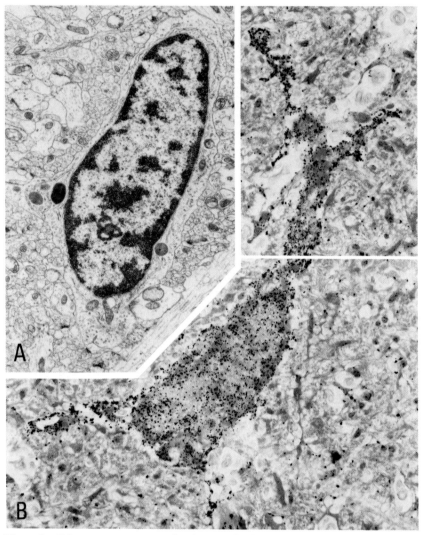

Fig. 6 Fine-structure of microglia in rabbit hippocampus
A: Conventional specimen. Nucleus is elongated and has large
blocks of heterochromatin. Cytoplasm shows long cisternae
of rough-surfaced endoplasmic reticulum and large dense
bodies. Note that the cytoplasmic matrix is electron lucent.
B: Silver carbonate stained microglia. Electron density of
this cell and of surrounding neuropil is high due to silver
deposit. Despite general high density, close examination
reveals fine-structural characteristics of this type of cell.

rence of this type of cells (Fig. 6A). This type of cells,
i.e., authentic microglial cells, made up 19% (31 out of 161
non-neuronal cells) of neuroglial cells in the stratum radiatum of rabbit hippocampus.

Morphology of the microglial cells is as follows. The nucleus
is elongated, irregular-shaped, but sometimes oval. It contains many blocks of heterochromatin and occasional nucleolus.
Perikaryal cytoplasm is scanty and extends into bipolar
processes. The contour of the cell shows spine-like projections jutting out at a right angle. In contrast to the silver
carbonate stained material, cytoplasmic matrix in conventional
electron micrographs appears pale. Microglial cells are not
dark cells. To the contrary, electron lucent cytoplasmic
matrix can be regarded as their characteristic feature of
the fine-structure (Fig. 6A). A few microtubules are detectable in glutaraldehyde-fixed specimens but no glial fibrils nor
glycogen particles are found. So we conclude that these are
the features of electron microscopic morphology of the microglial cells (Kitamura et al. 1977).

Difference from ologodendroglia

In contrast to the microglia described above, oligodendroglia
possess round or oval nucleus with large blocks of heterochromatin, located eccentrically at one pole of plump perikaryon. In the cytoplasm there are abundant ribosomes and microtubules oriented randomly. Cytoplasmic matrix is moderately
dense and sometimes appears fine granular. Cytoplasmic processes are thin and straight with abundant microtubules forming a bundle. These cells are identical with the dark oligodendroglia of Mori and Leblond (1970).

Difference from the transformed monocytes

In normal rabbit and mouse brains, cells with morphology of
monocytes or transformed monocytes are absent. In order to
elucidate differences from the monocytes in the nervous tissue, we examined rabbit brains with stab wounds made in the
hippocampal region. Around the stab wound, we could detect
many macrophages and their precursor cells. These transformed
monocytes are characterized with diffuse density in the cytoplasmic matrix, paucity of the ribosomes, blunt cytoplasmic
processes called ruffles, thin hyaloplasmic rims of the cytoplasm beneath the cell surface, and well developed endoplasmic reticulum and Golgi apparatus. The morphology is identical
with that of the transformed monocytes in the mouse brain
(Kitamura et al. 1972, Fujita and Kitamura 1976). Although
the nuclear shape and chromatin pattern resemble those of the
microglia, differences in the cytoplasmic features are clear
enough to distinguish both types of cells, even in pathologic-

al conditions. We came to a conclusion that the so-called
resting microglia or the microglia that are found in the normal adult brain are definitively different in morphology from
hematogenous cells, and constitute a distinct population
forming the third subspecies of neuroglia.

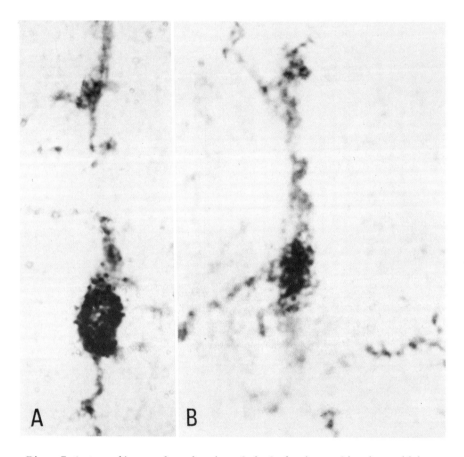

Fig. 7 Autoradiographs showing labeled microglia in rabbit
hippocampus, 39 hr after wounding. Specimens are stained by
silver carbonate method of Hortega, embedded in epoxy resin,
cut into semithin section and processed for ARG. ^{3}H-TdR is
given 2 hr prior to sacrifice. From A to D, the perikaryon
of a microglial cell becomes greatly enlarged and pale.
Finally (as in D), cell contour and cytoplasmic processes
become obscure and can only be seen by the presence of a
argyrophilic rim.

FUNCTION OF THE MICROGLIA

Till quite recently no one doubted the function of the microglia as a sole source of supply of brain macrophages. Therefore, it is no wonder that nothing appears left if this function of the microglia is absolutely denied as is done in the present work. A question should be asked anew, what is the function of microglia? In order to answer this question, we studied behavior of the microglia in reaction to brain injuries. To study dynamic pathology of the microglia, it was necessary to develop a technique of combination of the silver carbonate staining with ARG. It becomes feasible by using epon embedded semithin sections of impregnated materials

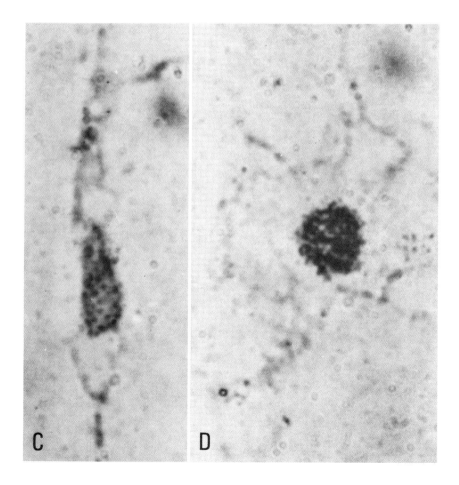

(Fujita and Kitamura 1974). ARG was performed on the semithin section. Metal salts used for the impregnation of the cells and tissues do not interfere with the processing of ARG since the specimens are wholly embedded in the epoxy resin and insulated from the photographic emulsion. Furthermore, this technique, as it uses the sections of 1 to 2 µm in thickness, has advantages of improving the resolution of the ARG significantly.

Reaction of the microglia in the rabbit hippocampus was studied by this technique together with EM and EM-ARG. It was found that as early as 24 hr after the stab wound, some microglial cells began to swell in cytoplasm and nucleus (Fig. 7).

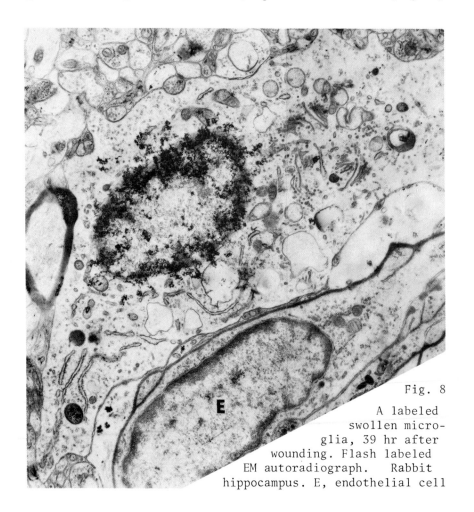

Fig. 8

A labeled swollen microglia, 39 hr after wounding. Flash labeled EM autoradiograph. Rabbit hippocampus. E, endothelial cell

The swelling was more marked in the perikaryon and proximal part of the cytoplasmic processes. Peripheral delicate processes tended to remain intact so that silver carbonate staining of the reactive microglia at this stage revealed typical microglial feature in the peripheral branching with swollen perikaryon (Fig. 7 A and B). Thirty-nine hours after stab wounding, the swelling of the microglial cells was found markedly advanced in many of them and 33% of the microglial cells in the stratum radiatum of hippocampus incorporated ^{3}H-TdR that was given 2 hr prior to sacrifice (Fig. 7). Most of their nuclei now became rounded and surrounded by a clear halo (Fig. 7 C and D). The very phenomenon has been called "acute swelling of oligodendroglia" by neuropathologists. It is beyond doubt that these figures are of reactive microglial cells, but not of oligodendroglial cells. Electron microscopic observation of these swollen microglia revealed that their intracytoplasmic organelles did not increase in proportion to the cytoplasmic swelling so that the cell body appeared very clear (Fig. 8). Some of the swollen microglia contained lipid droplets and a few microtubules. In contrast, oligodendroglia showed no morphological changes nor they began DNA synthesis. Astrocytes also showed very inconspicuous changes. Some of them became to contain glycogen particles but, other than this, their fine structure remained surprisingly unchanged. None of astrocytes in the rabbit hippocampus began to incorporate ^{3}H-TdR up to 39 hr after wounding. Only the microglia reacted to the brain injury by swelling and nuclear DNA synthesis. It is remarkable that, up to 39 hr after stab wounding, no oligodendroglia nor astrocytes responded with DNA synthesis as shown in Table 1.

Type of cells	Time after wounding		
	0 hr	30 hr	39 hr
Oligodendroglia	5	9 (0)	2 (0)
Immature astrocytes	12	9 (0)	5 (0)
Astrocytes	37	26 (0)	31 (0)
Microglia (swollen)	0	15(44)	18(33)
Microglia (resting)	10	0	2 (0)
Transformed monocytes	0	0	4 (0)

Table 1   Number of cells per 1 mm^2 of stratum radiatum of rabbit hippocampus, scored by EM-ARG. Percentages of labeled cells are shown in parentheses. Flash labeling.

It became clear that up to 39 hr after wounding only the microglia synthesized DNA. Based on this observation, we performed experiments to pursue metamorphosis and fate of the swollen microglia. First we made a stab wound in rabbit hippocampus, injected with ^{3}H-TdR locally 36 hr after wounding and killed the animals 3, 27 hr, 2.5, 6.5 and 12.5 days after the injection. Sections of the hippocampus were studied by ARG and occurrence of various kinds of neuroglial cells and labeling index of each cell type was counted. Results are shown in Table 2. As seen in Table 2, the ^{3}H-label did not appear on the astroglial nuclei until 2.5 days after the injection of ^{3}H-TdR. It is highly unlikely that the injected ^{3}H-TdR remained in the brain in an available form for more than 27 hr, so we concluded that the labeled astrocytes that first appeared 2.5 days after the injection should have come from non-astroglial precursors that had incorporated ^{3}H-TdR in earlier phases of the wound reaction. Oligodendroglia can not be the precursors since they did not incorporate ^{3}H-TdR throughout the experiment. The only candidate is the microglia. They had been already labeled in a high percentage immediately after the injection of ^{3}H-TdR (39 hr after wounding). It was evident that the microglia proliferated during this period but their number did not increase; 26 per 1 mm^2 at 27 hr after the injection (i.e. 63 hr after the injury) remained almost unchanged for next 1.5 days. It would be inconceivable that such an active proliferation of the microglial cells as indicated by 42% of the labeling index, resulted in no increase in cell number, unless we admit that newly produced daughter cells were constantly leaving the population. These newly formed cells should retain the label. And this label should be detectable in the cells that had changed from the

| Time after ^{3}H-Tdr | 3 hr | 27 hr | 2.5 | 6.5 | 12.5 days |
Time after injury	39 hr	63 hr	4	8	14 days
Oligodendroglia	2 (0)	2 (0)	1 (0)	6 (0)	5 (0)
Astroglia	31 (0) →	29 (0) →	45(11) →	84(75) →	166(68)
Microglia (reactive)	18(33) →	26(42) →	27(41) →	33(18) →	40(53)
Microglia (resting)	2 (0)				

Table 2 Number of cells per 1 mm^2 of stratum radiatum of rabbit hippocampus. A single injection of ^{3}H-TdR was given 36 hr after wounding. Labeling percentage of each cell type is shown in parentheses.

microglia. Having examined the results shown in Table 2, we concluded that some of the reactive microglia should have changed into astrocytes so that the astrocytes increased in number and in labeling percentage (cf. arrows in Table 1).

EM ARG taken at 8 and 14 post-traumatic days revealed presence of many labeled intermediate forms between swollen microglia and immature astrocytes, thereby corroborating the above conclusions of autoradiographic study. Finally they changed into cells that are characterized by bundles of glial filaments in the cytoplasm, glycogen particles, large dense bodies, many small vesicles, short rough-surfaced endoplasmic reticulum and swollen mitochondria. Nuclei are usually indented. We conclude that these organella-rich fibrous astrocytes with indented nucleus are transformed microglia (Fig. 9).

Transformation of the microglia into fibrous astrocytes in reaction to brain injuries implies an important function of the microglia to serve as reserve cells for the astrocytes.

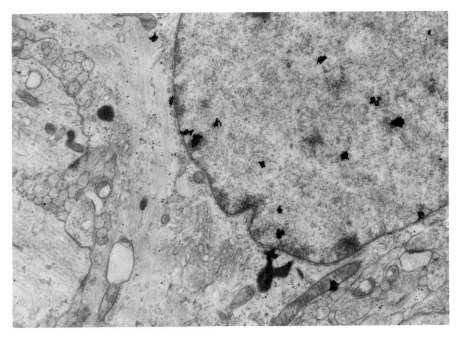

Fig. 9 Astroglial transformation of labeled microglia. 12.5 days after ^{3}H-TdR injection. The cell contains large bundles of glial filaments and is relatively rich in cell organelles.

Is transformation of Microglia into Fibrous Astrocytes a
General Phenomenon ?

We have concluded that the "resting" microglia in the
rabbit hippocampus proliferate from early phases of wound
reaction and change into fibrous astrocytes. A question
arises whether this phenomenon is peculiar to the microglia
of the rabbit hippocampus. We decided to investigate this
problem in the mouse brain. In order to study what kind of
cells are proliferating in the mouse brain immediately after
stab wounding and into what kind of cells they later change
we applied similar technique of pulse labeling with ^{3}H-TdR in
combination with EM and Cajal's gold sublimate staining. We
injected mice with ^{3}H-TdR repeatedly between 28 and 46 hr
after the stab wounding. Two mice each were sacrificed 2 hr
and 18 days after the final injection and the numbers of
labeled cells were counted on ARG of one whole frontal section of one mouse brain. At the same time, ratios of various
cell types were examined by EM ARG on another mouse and the
total number of labeled cells was alloted to each cell type.
Excepting the transformed monocytes, initial active proliferation was virtually restricted to microglia (Table 3).

A pair of mice received ^{3}H-TdR 34 hr after stab wounding
and were sacrificed 2 hr later to see what kind of cells were
proliferating. From one mouse, frozen sections were prepared
stained by Cajal's gold sublimate method, trimmed under a
microscope, embedded in epoxy resin, cut at 1∿2 μm and auto-
radiographed (Fig. 10). In these semithin sections, many
stained astrocytes were found but few of them showed silver
grains on their nuclei. Other than the transformed monocytes
that amounted to 80% of all the labeled cells, only small oval
nuclei surrounded by a clear halo were labeled. They were not

Time after ^{3}H-Tdr Time after injury	0 day 2 days		18 days 20 days	
Number of labeled cells in a frontal section	1035	→	226	
Type of labeled cells	(EM-ARG)		(EM-ARG)	
transformed monocytes	(37/46)	833	(6/106)	12
astrocytes	(1/46)	22 ⎫ 202	(88/106)	188 ⎫ 214
microglia	(8/46)	180 ⎭	(12/106)	26 ⎭

Table 3 Cells proliferating shortly after the stab wound
of the mouse brain and their fate.

stained by the gold sublimate method. Their morphology, reactive nuclear DNA synthesis, cytoplasmic swelling and unstain-
ability with the gold sublimate indicated that they are homologous to the reactive microglia of the rabbit hippocampus.
Observation by EM ARG on brain sections from another mouse
of the pair confirmed their characteristics of swollen microglia; the reactive DNA-synthetic cells were characterized by
a small oval nucleus with clumped chromatin blocks, shortened
stacks of rough-surfaced endoplasmic reticulum, small but
well developed Golgi apparatus, numerous small vesicles,

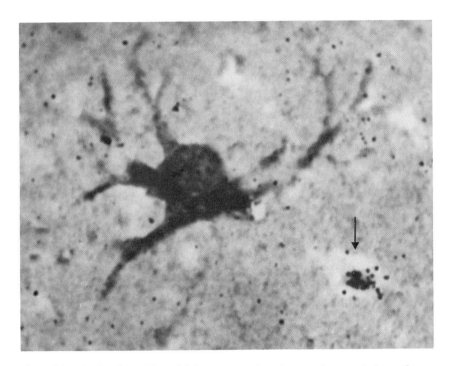

Fig. 10 ARG of gold sublimate stained specimen, taken from
one of the two mice that received ³H-TdR injection at 34 hr
after the wounding and were killed 2 hr later. Few of the
stained astrocytes incorporated ³H-TdR. Excepting transformed
monocytes, only small cells with oval nucleus (arrow) surrounded by a clear halo were labeled. Obviously they were non-astroglial cells. Reactive swelling of the cytoplasm and nuclear
DNA synthesis, together with morphological characteristics
suggested strongly that they are homologous cells of the
reactive microglia we have delineated in the rabbit brain.

occasional large dense bodies, a few microtubules, abundant
polysomes, presence of spine-like processes, swollen mitochondria and pale cytoplasmic matrix (Fig. 11). All these
features indicate that they belong to the microglial cells
in reactive state. Thus the situation was the same as in the
rabbit brain. Cells proliferating at early phases of reaction
to brain damage are the microglia and few astrocytes reacted
with DNA synthesis, if at all. The reactive microglia
also assume a typical figure of "acute swelling of oligodendroglia" in the mouse brain.

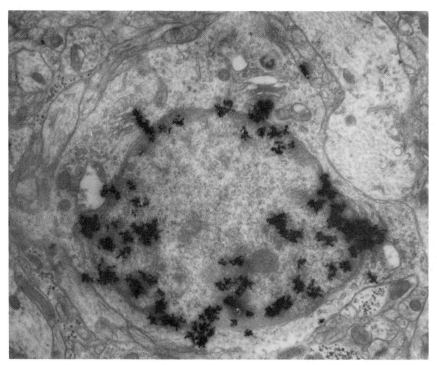

Fig. 11 EM ARG of brain of another mouse of the pair
described in legend of Fig. 10, fixed and processed for EM
ARG: ^{3}H-TdR was injected 34 hr after the wounding and the
animal was killed 2 hr later. Again astrocytes were not labeled. Excepting transformed monocytes, only the cells that are
morphologically homologous to the reactive microglia of the
rabbit hippocampus incorporated ^{3}H-TdR. These DNA-synthetic
cells were characterized by a small nucleus with many blocks
of clumped chromatin, numerous small vesicles, a few microtubules, spine-like processes, and pale cytoplasmic matrix.

In the brain of mice that survived 18 days more, i.e., killed at post-traumatic day 20, labeled cells were greatly reduced in number (from 1035 to 226, Table 3) but the majority of them now showed unmistakable characteristics of astrocytes, as shown in Figs. 12 and 13. They were rich in glial filaments and contained glycogen particles. Other cell organelles such as small vesicles and Golgi apparatus, short rough-surfaced endoplasmic reticulum, mitochondria were also relatively abundant. They had replaced the labeled reactive microglia that had proliferated 18 days before. In gold sublimate stain (Fig. 12), many astrocytes now showed ^{3}H-label and most of them were found to be fibrous and hypertrophied astrocytes. Results were again essentially the same as we observed in injured rabbit hippocampus.

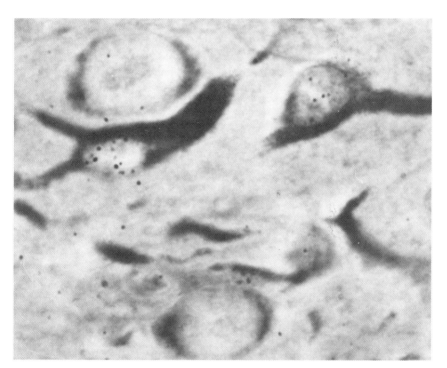

Fig. 12 ARG of gold sublimate stained specimen from one of two mice that received repeated injection of ^{3}H-TdR between 28 and 46 hr after the stab wounding and survived further 18 days. Numerous hypertrophied fibrous astrocytes now showed nuclear labeling with ^{3}H-TdR, thereby indicating that they were transformed from the reactive microglia.

We came to conclusions that:
(1) In the mouse brain as well, the microglia proliferate in the earliest in response to stab wound and later transform into reactive, fibrous, hypertrophied astrocytes. The pattern of the reaction is essentially the same as we observed in the stratum radiatum of rabbit hippocampus.
(2) It is likely that the microglia serve as reserve cells for astrocytes in adult brains of mouse and rabbit.
(3) It seems right to generalize these conclusions, since the same phenomenon is repeatedly observed in mouse and rabbit brains.
(4) The function of the microglia, so far as we could uncover, is to proliferate in response to the brain injury and to repair the damage of the nervous tissue by producing astro-

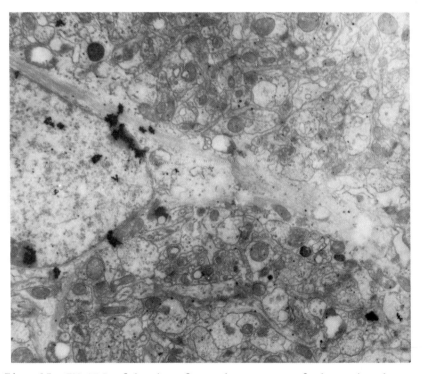

Fig. 13   EM ARG of brain of another mouse of the pair that are described in legend of Fig. 12: Labeled cumulatively between 28 and 46 post-traumatic hours and survived 18 days more. Most of the labeled cells now contained bundles of glial filaments and glycogen particles.

cytosis and astrogliosis.

(5) In EM ARG, we could differentiate transformed monocytes and macrophages from the reactive microglia, although both were labeled in earlier stages of wound reaction. They are different in origin, morphology and function.

GENERAL CONCLUSIONS AND SUMMARY

1. There has been considerable confusion in use of the term "microglia". It is mainly, I believe, due to semantic errors of calling transformed monocytes and the resting microglia by the same name of "microglia". To avoid this confusion, the name "microglia" should be used only for the "resting" microglia that are present in the normal adult brain and those that are proved to be directly related to the "resting" microglia. Transformed monocytes and brain macrophages should not be called "microglia".

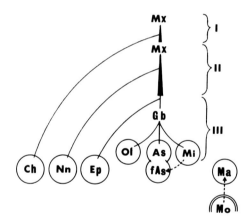

Fig. 14 Schematic representation of histogenesis of the microglia and other kinds of cells from matrix cells. Arrows with interrupted lines indicate cellular transformation in pathological conditions. Mx represents matrix cells; Gb, glioblasts; Ch, choroid plexus epithelium; Nn, neurons; Ep, ependymal cells; Ol, oligodendroglia; As, astroglia; fAs, fibrous astrocytes; Mi, microglia; Mo, circulating blood monocytes; Ma, brain macrophages. I, II and III indicate stage I, II and III of cytogenesis of the CNS, respectively.

2. The microglia are the third subspecies of neuroglia, as their name "micro-*glia*" represents. They are differentiated from glioblasts at the third stage of cytogenesis of the CNS (cf. Fig. 14).

3. The microglia can be identified in its resting form by electron microscopy as cells having distinctive morphological characteristics.

4. The microglia are the cells that react in the earliest to damages of the CNS with their cytoplasmic swelling and nuclear DNA synthesis. The nucleus becomes oval or rounded. The reactive microglia frequently assume a form of small round cell with a spherical nucleus surrounded by a clear halo. Neuropathologists have called them "acute swelling of oligodendroglia".

5. The microglia, after the reactive proliferation, change into fibrous astrocytes (Fig. 9, 12, 13 and 14).

6. One function of the microglia, so far uncovered, is to serve as reserve cells for astroglia in the adult CNS and to contribute to astrocytosis and astrogliosis in pathological conditions.

7. It was reconfirmed, by immunohistochemical studies, that the microglia are unrelated to the macrophage system, and that the brain macrophages are derived from circulating monocytes (cf. Fig. 3, 4 and 14).

As a schematic representation of the general conclusions the histogenetic place and the function of the microglia are shown in a summarized form in Fig. 14.

REFERENCES

Baringer JR, Griffith JF (1970). Experimental herpes simplex encephalitis: Early neuropathologic changes. J Neuropath exp Neurol 29:89-104.

Del Rio-Hortega P (1919). El tercer elemento de los centros nerviosos. I. La microglia en estado normal. II. Intervención de la microglia en los processos patologicos. (Celulas en bastoncito y cuerpos granulo-adiposos). III. Naturaleza probable de la microglia. Bol Soc Esp Biol 9:68-120.

Del Rio-Hortega P (1921). Histogenesis y evolucion normal; exodo y distribucion regional de la microglia. Arch Neuro-biol 2:212-255.

Del Rio-Hortega P (1932). Microglia. In Penfield W (ed): "Cytology and Cellular Pathology of the Nervous System,"

Vol. 2, New York: Hoeber,p 482-534.

Field EJ, Raine CS (1969). Experimental allergic encephalo-myelitis in the rhesus monkey. J Neurol Sci 8:379-411.

Fujita H, Fujita S (1964). Electron microscopic studies on the differentiation of the ependymal cells and the glio-blasts in the spinal cord of domestic fowl. Z Zellforsch 64:262-272.

Fujita S (1963). The matrix cell and cytogenesis in the developing central nervous system. J comp Neurol 120:37-42.

Fujita S (1964). Analysis of neuron differentiation in the central nervous system by tritiated thymidine autoradio-graphy. J comp Neurol 122:311-328.

Fujita S (1965). An autoradiographic study on the origin and fate of the sub-pial glioblasts in the embryonic chick spinal cord. J comp Neurol 124:51-60

Fujita S (1966) Application of light and electron microscopic autoradiography to the study of cytogenesis of the fore-brain. In Hassler R, Stephan H (ed): "Evolution of the Forebrain", Stuttgart: Thieme, p 180-196.

Fujita S (1973) Genesis of glioblast in the human spinal cord as revealed by Feulgen cytophotometry. J comp Neurol 151: 25-34

Fujita S, Kitamura T (1974) Origin and fate of reactive neuroglia in the damaged mouse brain—Transformation of oligodendroglia to astrocytes—. Abstracts of VII Intern Congr Neuropath, Budapest, p 95.

Fujita S, Kitamura T (1975). Origin of brain macrophages and the nature of the so-called microglia. Acta neuropath Suppl 4:291-296.

Fujita S, Kitamura T (1976). Origin of brain macrophages and the nature of the microglia. In Zimmerman HM (ed): "Progr-ess in Neuropathology,"vol 3, New York, Grune & Stratton, p 1-50.

Fujita S, Tsuchihashi Y, Kitamura T (1978). Absence of hemato-genous cells in the normal brain parenchyma as revealed by anti-leukocytic antibody. J Neuropath exp Neurol 37:615.

Hattori H (1973). EM-autoradiographic studies on the origin, nature and fate of reactive cells in the central nervous system of mouse after stab-wounding. J Kyoto Pref Univ Med 82:1-24.

His W (1889). Die Neuroblasten und deren Entstehung im embryo-nalen Mark. Arch Anat Physiol 5:249-300.

Kitamura T, Hattori H, Fujita S (1972). Autoradiographic stud-ies on histogenesis of brain macrophages in the mouse. J Neuropath exp Neurol 31:502-518.

Kitamura T, Hattori H, Fujita S (1973). EM-autoradiographic

studies on the inflammatory cells in the experimental Japanese encephalitis. J Electron Microsc 21:315-322.

Kitamura T, Tsuchihashi Y, Tatebe A, Fujita S (1977). Electron microscopic features of the resting microglia in the rabbit hippocampus, identified by silver carbonate staining. Acta neuropath 38:195-201.

Kitamura T, Tsuchihashi Y, Fujita S (1978). Initial response of silver-impregnated "resting microglia" to stab wounding in rabbit hippocampus. Acta neuropath 44:31-39.

Lampert P (1967). Electron microscopic studies on ordinary and hyperacute experimental allergic encephalomyelitis. Acta neuropath 9:99-126.

Mori S, Leblond CP (1969). Identification of microglia in light and electron microscopy. J comp Neurol 125:57-80.

Mori S, Leblond CP (1970). Electron microscopic identification of three classes of oligodendroglia and a preliminary study of their proliferative activity in the corpus callosum of young rats. J comp Neurol 139:1-30.

Oehmichen M, Wiethölter H, Graeves M (1979). Immunological analysis of human microglia: Lack of monocytic and lymphoid membrane differentiation antigens. J Neuropath exp Neurol 38:99-103.

Penfield W (1932). Neuroglia: Normal and Pathological. In Penfield W (ed): "Cytology and Cellular Pathology of the Nervous System,: New York, Hoeber, p 422-479.

Persson LI, Rönnbäck L, Rosengren LE (1978). Identification of reactive cells in the injured brain. Acta neurol Scand 57, Suppl 67:245-246.

Prineas J, Raine CS, Wisnewski H (1969). An ultrastructural study of experimental demyelination and remyelination. Part III. Chronic experimental allergic encephalomyelitis in the central nervous system. Lab Invest 21:472-483.

Ramon y Cajal S (1908). Nouvelles observations sur l'évolution des neuroblasts, avec quelques remarques sur l'hypothése neurogénétique de Hensen-Held. Anat Anz 32:1-25, 65-87.

Ramon y Cajal S (1920). Algunas consideraciones sobre la mesoglia de Roberston y Rio-Hortega. Trab Lab Invest Biol Univ Madrid 18:109-127.

Sato M (1968). ^{3}H-Thymidine autoradiographic studies on the origin of reactive cells in the brain of mice infected with Japanese encephalitis virus. Brain Nerve (Tokyo) 20:1239-1250 (In Japanese with English abstract).

Tsuchihashi Y, Kitamura T, Fujita S (1977). Immunohistochemical studies on the brain macrophages and the so-called amoeboid microglia. Igaku no Ayumi (Tokyo) 103:517-518 (In Japanese).

Unanue ER (1968). Properties and some uses of anti-macrophage antibodies. Nature 218:36-38.

Wood GW, Gollahan K, Tilzer SA, Vars T, Morantz RA (1979). The failure of microglia in normal brain to exhibit mononuclear phagocyte markers. J Neuropath exp Neurol 38: 369-376.

Eleventh International Congress of Anatomy:
Glial and Neuronal Cell Biology, pages 171–185

MICROGLIA IN THE HUMAN CORTEX: AN ULTRASTRUCTURAL STUDY

Jean-Francois Foncin

Ecole Pratique des Hautes Etudes and Unite 106,
I.N.S.E.R.M. Laboratoire Montyon
LaSalpêtrière, F75651 Paris, Cedex 13, France

1.   INTRODUCTION

Ultrastructural study of microglia in humans runs into
two difficulties: In common with all neuromorphological
endeavours in our species, experimentation is impossible, and
the basis of research is observational data, often gathered
more through luck than through design.   Particularly in the
case of human microglia, nuclear isotopic labeling data are
unavailable, even though this technique in other species is
the basis of important arguments pertaining to origin and
evolution, (Adrian and Walker, 1962; Konigsmar and Sidman,
1963), as well as the source of much controversy (Adrian and
Schelper, this volume).

In spite of these restrictions, such studies must be
undertaken: First, there are considerable species differences
in mammals in the appearance and behavior of microglia and one
knows that it is not by chance that Hortega's classical paper
used the rabbit as a source of material for illustrations
(Hortega, 1921, 1954).   Second, the variety of pathological
conditions open to observation in the human enables us to
observe, without undue influence by a priori hypotheses, a
whole range of reaction modalities.   Needless to say, we are
more often led to inferences than to demonstrations. Third,
study of microglia in the human is necessary if we hope for
eventual relevance to medical application.

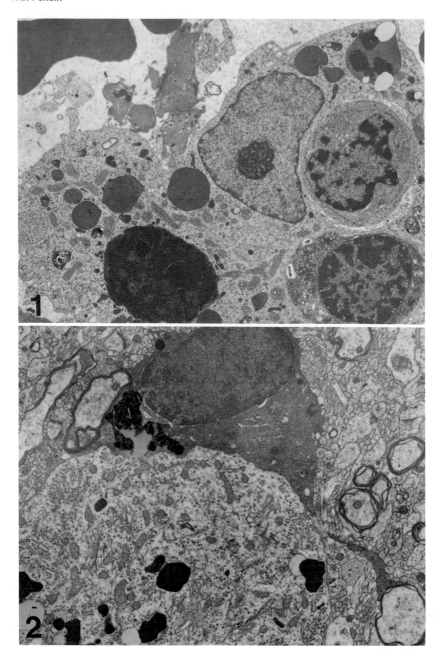

II. MATERIALS AND METHODS

Material used for the present study was obtained in the course of neurosurgical operations, either curative or exploratory in purpose, mainly in the Neurosurgical Unit of the Salpêtrière, Paris in the years 1964 to 1978. It was selected from about 1,000 specimens, representing various conditions affecting the brain in the adult. Specimens were taken with a sharp No. 4 curette, and immediately immersed in 5% glutaraldehyde or glutaraldehyde-paraformaldehyde mixture according to Karnowsky, with phosphate buffer. After fixation they were transferred into the same buffer with 0.2 M sucrose added. They remained in the buffer for a variable time, the duration of which did not appear to influence the results. Fixed specimens were cut into pieces less than 1 mm across, postfixed in osmium tetroxide without block staining, embedded in Araldite, and stained with uranyl acetate and lead citrate on thin sections.

Our material originated from pathological subjects. Nevertheless, some figures may be considered as representative of the normal, in particular those obtained at a distance from any lesion or those obtained during psychosurgery for intractable pain.

III RESULTS

The idea could be entertained, that ideal material for the study of microglia in the human would result from the pure proliferation of the line: "microgliomatosis" as described by D. Russel (1948) and others. In fact, electron microscope studies have shown that this tumor type should be classified in the lymphoma group. The problem is further complicated, and previous interpretations of this tumor explained, by the importance of reactive phenomena in the midst of lymphoid proliferation (Fig. 1). Many cells with cytoplasmic characteristics akin to those of "reactive microglia" phagocytose tumor cells; it is possible that selective impreg-

---

Fig. 1 Primitive brain lymphoma. Macrophage is engulfing lymphoma cells. x 11000

Fig. 2 Frontal topectomy for intractable pain. Satellite oligodendrocyte. Note a process arising most probably from the same cell and reaching to myelin sheath. x 7600

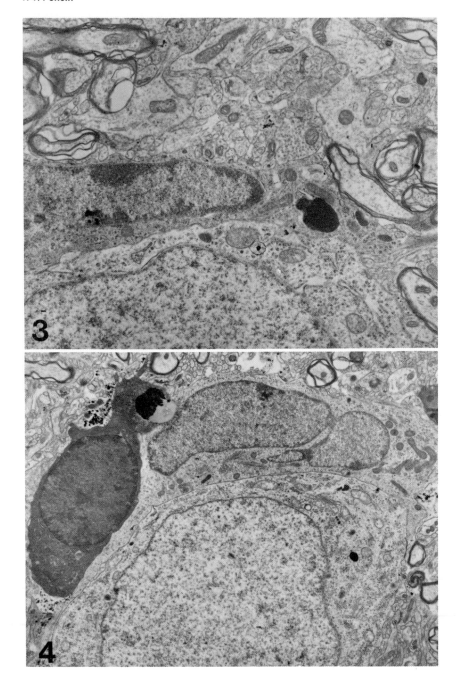

nation of these cells with silver techniques led to the attribution of the whole tumor to the microglia line. At any rate, useful discussion of the possible autochthonous or allochthonous origin of these tumor cells cannot be based on such differentiated cells.

Satellite Microglia

The majority of satellite cells to be found around neuronal perikarya are undoubedly related to oligodendroglia (Fig. 2) as characterized by their cytoplasm with clear cisternae standing out against a dark background, and their ellipsoid nucleus with uniform chromatin; in rare instances, demonstration is provided by the occurrence of a cytoplasmic process containing tubules and extended to a myelin sheath. This type of cell may contain dense inclusions of the lysosome type, as do many interfascicular oligodendrocytes; consequently, the occurrence of inclusions does not indicate the microglial nature of any given brain cell. In "normal" human cortex, however, satellite cells are found which differ notably from oligodendrocytes and from the exceptional satellite astrocytes. Their nucleus is more elongated, and less dense, with marginated chromatin. The cytoplasm is clearer than that of the above described cells. It often reaches farther along the neuron plasma membrane than in the cells of the first type. It contains numerous ribosomes in rosette arrangement, mitochondria with a denser matrix, no tubules, and dense bodies of the lysosome type, often of a more polymorphous character than in the first group (Fig. 3).

The modifications in structure and outline of this latter cell type (microglia) were studied under pathological conditions. The nucleus is clearer, with clear-cut marginated chromatin; a nucleolus is often prominent. In the cytoplasm, ergastoplasm is organized into lamellar structures, but, at least in the early stages, these changes are not

---

Fig. 3.   Satellite microglia in the normal; compare with Fig. 2. x 14700.
Fig. 4.   Cortex at a distance from a corpus callosum tumor. A nerve cell shows dispersed ribosomes; retrograde reaction? The dark cell (oligodendrocyte) is separated from the nerve cell by the cytoplasm of a reactive microglial cell which stretches out on more than a third of the nerve cell circumference.   x 5100

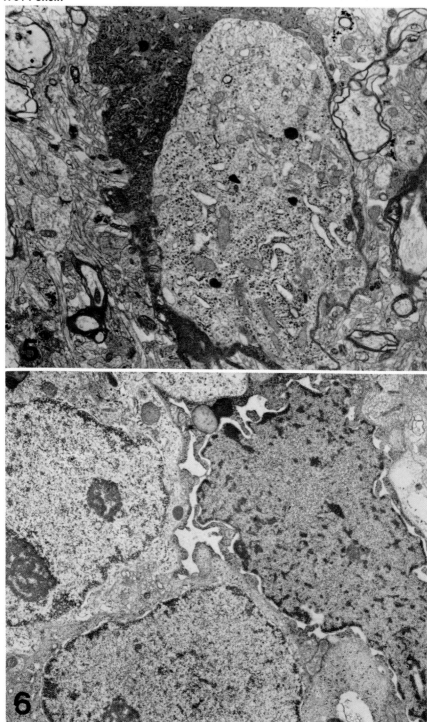

See legends, page 178.

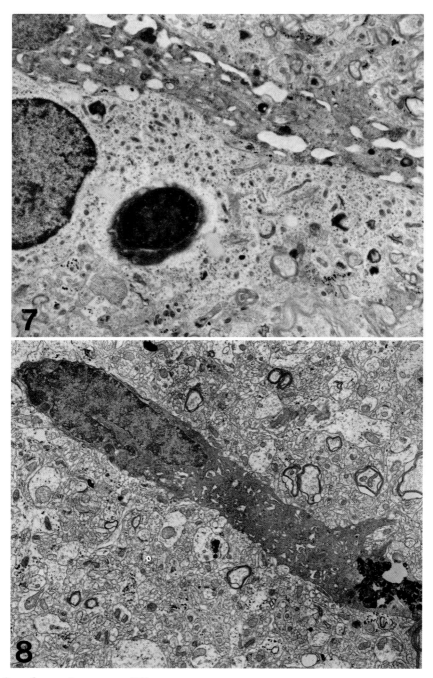

See legends, page 178.

striking. The outline of the cell, on the contrary, is con-
spicuously modified as a result of an extension of microglial
cell processes around the nerve cell. They isolate the latter
not only from presynaptic terminals, as shown by Blinzinger
and Kreutzberg, (1968) in the course of experimental retrograde reaction, but from satellite oligodendroglial cells as
well (Fig. 4), demonstrating the distinction between the two
cell types. This kind of microglial reaction corresponds to
moderate changes in the neuron, as may be observed in the
cortex in the vicinity of deep tumors. Even in those cases,
the neuron perikaryon may be almost completely separated from
the neuropile, at least in a given plane of section, by a
thin layer of microglial cytoplasm (Fig. 5). When neuron
lesions are more marked, microglia are organized around the
nerve cell in a nodular fashion; ten years ago, we considered
this type of nodule of oligodendrogial origin (Foncin, 1970).
In fact, the characteristics of the nodular cells themselves,
as described at that time (relatively clear cytoplasm, ribosome arrangement in rosettes, dense mitochondria, nucleolated
nucleus), as well as the later observation of intermediate
forms, show that, at least in a number of instances, and in
particular in the case illustrated at that time, these nodules
are really, as postulated by classical neuropathology, of
microglial origin (Fig. 6). In the course of further evolution, when the nerve cell is reduced to a retracted skel-
eton, an occasional altered oligodendrocyte may be seen en-
gulfed in an hypertrophied microglial cell (Fig.7).

Fig. 5. Late post-traumatic dementia. A nerve cell is almost completely isolated by microglial processes. x 10000
Fig. 6. Chronic thrombosis of the superior sagittal sinus.
A microglial nodule surrounds a nerve cell showing chronic
ischemic lesion. x 11400
Fig. 7. Hexachlorophene intoxication. Part of a retracted
and profoundly altered nerve cell. A microglial cell is
considerably hypertrophied and engulfs a pycnotic cell,
probable remnant of satellite oligodendrocyte. x 7400
Fig. 8. At a distance from an intracerebral hematoma, an
elongated cell with thorny processes and lysosome-like inclusions shows, nevertheless, cytoplasmic characteristics
of oligodendroglia. x 6700

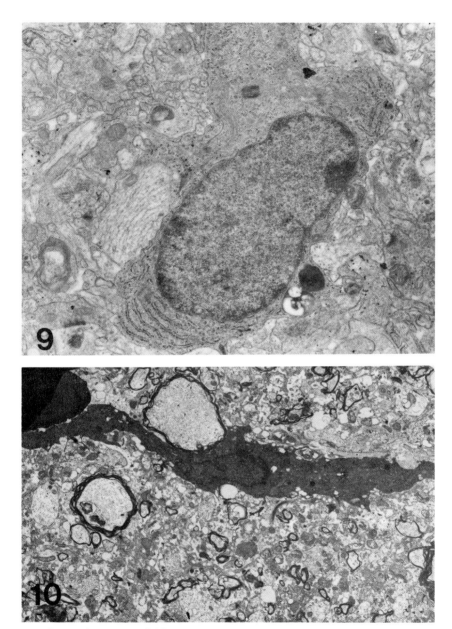

See legends, page 180.

Interstitial Microglia

Contrary to satellite microglia, human interstitial
microglia, at least in our experience, have proven difficult
or impossible to identify in the normal. We did not find
"microglia" cells that could be distinguished with any cer-
tainty from interfascicular oligodendroglia within the static
electronmicroscope picture of normal cortex or white matter.
Even in pathological instances, cells which evidently appear
to be in the course of a mobilizing process, with an elongated outline and spiny appendages (Fig. 8), show characteristics of the oligodendroglia line, such as homogenous nucleus and dark cytoplasm with clear cisternae. Even the presence of lysosomal inclusions, which could be interpreted
as evidence of macrophage activity, is not a sure landmark of
microglial origin, as already noted concerning satellite
cells. Reactive cells corresponding to microglia, as usually
identified with the light microscope, often have a darker
cytoplasm than that of satellite microglia. Nevertheless,
the above-mentioned dense mitochondria and ribosome rosettes
may be found in these cells. In some instances the ergastoplasm is organized in parallel cisternae (Fig. 9), to such an
extent that the cell may be difficult to distinguish from a
fibroblast. On the other hand, rod cells, unequivoqual
equivalent of those described with the light microscope in
classical neuropathology, are found in numerous instances of
subacute or chronic disease; correspondence between light and
electronmicroscope images is evident and does not warrant the
use of "specific metallic" impregnation. A very elongated
nucleus, with dense marginated chromatin, a very elongated
cell body, with dense cytoplasm isolated ribosomes or short
ergastoplasmic cisternae concur in the description (Fig. 10).
Cell processes are short, at least in a given plane of section, and often take off perpendicularly from the long axis of
the cell; they appear to find their way between elements of
the neuropile. The thorny appearance of rod microglia in
silver light microscopic preparations seems to correspond to
a passive moulding or negative image of pre-existing elements.
Frequently, cell processes, mainly those situated at a distance from the nucleus, form short vela and tend to engulf

---

Fig. 9. "Pseudotumor cerebri". Probably microglial cell,
with mild reactive signs. x 14400
Fig. 10. Vicinity of metastatic melanoma. Rod microglia,
with part of an unmodified oligodendrocyte. x 2550

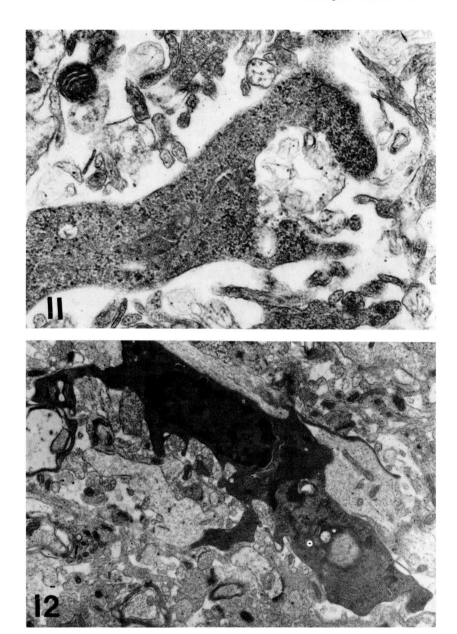

See legends, page 182.

adjacent elements, even when the latter are not morphologically altered. Passage from microglia-like cells to macrophages could be inferred from such images (Fig. 11). Nevertheless, as we will discuss later, it is by no means established that a majority of macrophages observed in the central nervous system are derived from microglial cells as
above described. The ultrastructural appearance of brain
macrophages is both unspecific and polymorphous. Their
nucleus is rounded or more or less indented; the cytoplasm
is laden with inclusions and contains short ergastoplasmic
cisternae; it sends out thin infolded vela which engulf cellular elements, necrotic debris or extracellular protein-
laden fluid, as objects of the macrophaging process. Detailed study of these cells would be outside the scope of
this paper because, even if some of them were derived from
microglia, they cannot be recognized morphologically as such
(Figs. 12 and 13).

IV   DISCUSSION

The first level of discussion is concerned with the
morphological definition of microglia at the ultrastructural
level. A "taxonomic" attitude would be to start from the
definition of the species by the original author, and to
transpose it to the electron microscope scale through the
study of thin sections of material impregnated according to
Hortega's methods. That is the purpose of the classical
paper by Mori and Leblond (1969). In fact, the cells we
describe as satellite microglia in the normal have many land-
marks in common with the cells identified as microglia by
these authors with the aid of a comparison of both techniques.

Our biopsy material is necessarily small in volume; it
is fixed under conditions optimal for electron microscopy,
and not for silver impregnation; moreover, a single multi-
purpose technique was indicated, in view of the many problems
under investigation. Comparison of impregnated and standard
material was not done, and we adopted for microglia a defini-

---

Fig. 11.   Encephalitis (benign outcome, undetermined agent).
Apparent macrophagic activity of the extremity of a rod cell
in altered neuropile.   x 50400
Fig. 12.   Tuberculous meningitis.   Beginning of macrophagic
transformation.   x 10800

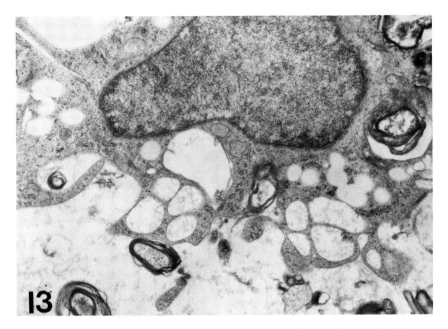

Fig. 13. Acute hemorrhagic leucoencephalitis (Hurst). Undeterminate macrophage. x 14400

tion by exclusion, in the way originally followed by the Spanish school; "el tercer elemento". One should bear in mind, nevertheless, that this expression does not correspond to the same object according to Cajal and to Hortega (the reader is referred to Hortega, 1921, 1954). According to Cajal neuron and astrocyte constitute the two first elements, and oligodendroglia and microglia are lumped together into the third one, according to Hortega neuron and (astro- + oligodendro-) glia constitute the two first elements, and microglia the third one.

Peters et al.(1970) reviewed a number of papers, the authors of which proceeded by elimination to attribute to microglia those cells which could not be classified as neuron, astrocyte or oligodendrocyte. There is a risk, proceeding that way, of lumping together into microglia various cells which could not be identified as a result of artefacts, especially after immersion fixation. We feel, however, that long experience in evaluating diverse material now allows a firm judgement; the possibility seems remote to mistake arte-

factually dark nerve cells for microglia (Peters et al.,).
A certain ambiguity was introduced by Vaughn and Peters (1968),
according to whom in the adult rat a "third type" of glial
cell constitutes a precursor pool. As described by these
authors, this cell appears to be identical with the satellite
microglial cell as above described; nevertheless, contrary
to these authors, we did not observe the sheet of astrocyte
cytoplasm interposed between microglia and neuron that they
consider a characteristic of that type of cell.

The second point of discussion relates to the evolution
of microglia under the influence of various agents. Due to
the many pathologic factors concerned, our material lends
itself to such a study; but it remains difficult to infer a
sequence of events from a mere juxtaposition of images. We
need the data from nuclear labeling, or even data from the
mitosis counts made possible by the observation of a large
number of cells under the light microscope (Cammermeyer,
1970). Concerning satellite microglia, however, we are able
to identify such cells in the normal, and to follow their
modifications step by step. The reactive satellites do
appear to be autochthonous, and the views of Fujita and
Kitamura (1976, p. 28) do not apply in our settings. On the
contrary, concerning interfascicular microglia, the difficulty in establishing a distinction, in the normal, between
oligodendrocytes and possible microgliocytes is depriving
us of a firm starting base. We evidently cannot bring new
viewpoints to a discussion which is centered on the autochthonous vs exogenous origin of reactive cells, and which
revolves around the reliability of isotope nuclear labeling.
Fujita and Kitamura, while proposing an exogenous origin for
all macrophages, do admit an autochthonous, microglial affiliation of the rod cells found, for instance, in cases of
general paresis. The ultrastructural counterpart of such
cells is certainly to be found in the "microglia" as described above. We have shown that rod cells exhibit macrophagic properties; from that fact we cannot draw conclusions
concerning the origin of macrophages in general.

V   CONCLUSION

Ultrastructural study of human cerebral cortex allows
us to define: 1. Satellite microglia in the normal, and
its evolution concomitant with neuron changes; 2. Interfascicular rod microglia, which exhibit macrophage properties.

The counterpart of the latter cell in the normal, as well as its subsequent evolution and the origin of most brain macrophages, remains as yet undetermined.

Acknowledgements

We wish to thank Mme Perre (C.N.R.S.) (microscopy and bibliography), M. Le Cren (I.N.S.E.R.M.) (photography) and Mme de Grolier (secretarial help). Supported in part by I.N.S.E.R.M., A.R.S. No. 6.

REFERENCES

Adrian EK, Walker BE (1962). Incorporation of thymidine H^3 by cells in normal and injured mouse spinal cord. J Neuropath Exp Neurol 21: 579-609.

Blinzinger K, Kreutzberg GW (1968). Displacement of synaptic terminals from regenerating motoneurons by microglial cells. Z Zellforsch 85: 145-157.

Cammermeyer J (1970). A light microscopic study of microglial cells: mitosis, development and proliferation. Masson (ed): VIth Congress Int Neuropathology Paris pp. 424-436.

Foncin JF (1970). Pathologie ultrastructurale de la glie chez l'homme. Masson (ed): VIe Congrès International de Neuropathologie Paris pp. 377-391.

Fujita S, Kitamura T (1976). Origin of brain macrophages and the nature of the microglia. In Zimmermann HM (ed) Progress in neuropathology vol III Grune and Stratton, London p. 1.

Hortega Del Rio P (1921). Histogenesis y evolucion normal: exodo y distribucion regional de la microglia. Memorias de la Real Sociedad espanola de historia natural Tome XI pp. 213.

Hortega Del Rio P (1954). Histogenesis y evolucion normal: exodo y distribucion regional de la microglia. Archivos de Histologia normal y pathologica, Buenos Aires V pp. 105-150.

Konigsmark BW, Sidman RL (1963). Origin of brain macrophages in the mouse. J Neuropath Exp Neurol 22: 643-676.

Mori S, Leblond CP (1969). Identification of microglia in light and electron microscopy. J Comp Neurol 135: 57-80.

Russel DS, Marshall AME, Smith FB (1948). Microgliomatosis (a form of reticulosis affecting the brain). Brain 71: 1-15.

Eleventh International Congress of Anatomy:
Glial and Neuronal Cell Biology, pages 187—196
© **1981 Alan R. Liss, Inc., 150 Fifth Avenue, New York, NY 10011**

ACCUMULATION OF 14C-5,6-DIHYDROXYTRYPTAMINE-MELANIN IN
INTRATHECAL AND SUBEPENDYMAL PHAGOCYTES OF THE RAT CNS AND
POSSIBLE ROUTES OF THEIR ELIMINATION FROM BRAIN

H.G.Baumgarten, F. Moritz and H.G.Schlossberger

Department of Neuroanatomy and Electron Microscopy, Free University of Berlin, Berlin-West
Max-Planck-Institute for Biochemistry, Martinsried, GFR

SUMMARY

14C-5,6-DHT-Melanin, a labelled synthetic polymer resembling the naturally occurring melanin formed in brain by autoxidation of dopamine, was injected into the left lateral ventricle of adult rats, and its fate followed by autoradiography and by transmission electron microscopy of structures
identified as labelled in preceding light micrographs, and
by EM-autoradiography.Shortly after injection, melanin particles (easily identified in the em because of their size,
structure and electron opacity) were seen ingested by supraependymal and epiplexus cells, by cells residing in the pia-
arachnoid, i.e. free subarachnoidal cells and perivascular
cells, and by subependymally located microglia-like cells
with intraventricular processes. Up to day four, an increase
in the number of labelled phagocytes in the CSF was noted
which transformed into typical reactive macrophages. Beyond
this time, many intraventricular melanin-loaded phagocytes
formed rounded clusters; cells of such clusters were subsequently found to invade the brain parenchyma by penetrating
the ependymal lining and to accumulate in the perivascular
space of brain vessels.14C-Melanin-storing macrophages were
found in the marginal sinus of the deep jugular lymph nodes
suggesting emigration of CNS-derived phagocytes via lymphatics or prelymphatics that contact the subarachnoidal space
compartment. This does not exclude the possibility that some
of the macrophages leave the brain via the systemic circulation by penetrating the vascular endothelium; these may be
disposed of in peripheral organs other than the lymph nodes.

The ability of supraependymal, epiplexus, free subarachnoidal and perivascular cells in the pia and of subependymal microglia cells to accumulate synthetic melanin by phagocytosis suggests that these cells are local variants of the same type of resting potential phagocytes of the mammalian brain.

The CSF appears to be replenished with phagocytes by mitosis and migration of microglia-like cells or their precursors located underneath the ependyma of the lateral ventricle and by mitosis of resting intrathecal cells.

MATERIAL AND METHODS

14C-5,6-dihydroxytryptamine-melanin was prepared from 5,6-dihydroxytryptamine (5,6-DHT) by autoxidation at pH 8; 20 μl of a melanin-containing suspension (corresponding to 50 /g free base 14C-5,6-DHT) was injected into the left lateral ventricle of ether anaesthetized rats. The rats were killed at various intervals after injection (1 h up to 14 days) and the animals fixed by intracardiac infusion of glutaraldehyde. The brain, deep jugular lymph nodes, spleen, kidneys and lungs were removed from the animals and slices from these organs prepared by hand; the slices were then postfixed in OsO_4, dehydrated and embedded in Epon 812. Semithin sections and ultrathin sections were prepared for either routine light and electron microscopic analysis or for light and elctron microscopic autoradiography (for details of the techniques used, see Moritz et al. 1980). Structures identified as radiolabelled in light microscopic autoradiograms were generally analyzed for ultrastructural details in consecutive ultrathin sections by TEM .

RESULTS AND DISCUSSION

Soon after injection, melanin particle aggregates (cf.Fig. 1,2) were either observed in the lumen of the

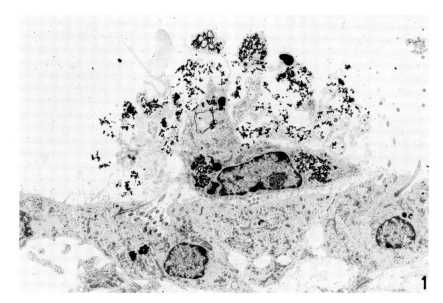

Fig. 1:
Intraventricularly located supraependymal cell actively involved in accumulating melanin particles by phagocytosis.
Note extracellular melanin particle aggregates. 24 h after
14C-5,6-DHT-melanin injection. x 2960

lateral ventricles without recognizable relation to cells or
cell processes or confined to processes of supraependymal
(Fig. 1) and epiplexus cells as well as intraventricular processes of subependymal microglia-like cells (Fig. 3). The
particulate polymer was taken up into the cells by phagocytosis vacuoles (cf. Fig. 1) and, in later stages, incorporated into phagosomes. Already by six h after injection, melanin-loaded cells were detected in the basal cisterns of
the CSF (free subarachnoidal cells and perivascular cells).
Following phagocytic uptake of large amounts of 14C-5,6-
DHT-melanin, the cells transformed into typical rounded reactive macrophages. By four days after injection, many supraependymal phagocytes tended to form large rounded clusters,were subsequently found to invade the brain parenchyma (Fig. 2) and to migrate towards subependymally located
vessels. After invading the brain matter (Fig. 5,6), some
cells showed typical features of reactive microglia-like

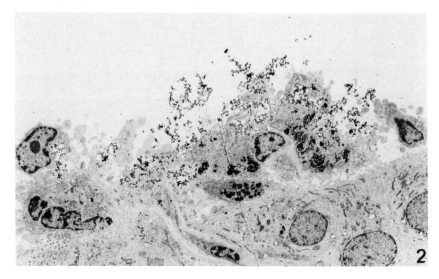

Fig. 2:
Cluster of supraependymal cells involved in accumulation of
melanin. Note penetration of one cell of this cluster into
the subependymal neuropil; this cell has microglia-like
features. 4 days after 14C-5,6-DHT melanin. x 2960

cells (Fig. 2) and, later on, of macrophages (i.e. when they
approached the brain vessels). Between day one and two, many
unlabelled microglia-like cells were detected underneath
the ependyma of the lateral ventricle and many cells in the
subependymal layer were noted to undergo mitosis (Fig. 4).
The transformation of subependymal cells into various types
of glial cells including microglia has previously been demonstrated by thymidine autoradiography (Paterson et al.
1973) confirming the results presented here. Infrequently,
intrathecal cells were also noted to undergo mitotic divisions. Melanin-loaded macrophages appeared to leave the
subarachnoidal space either via blood vessels or via lymphatics (or prelymphatics) since they were found in the marginal sinuses of the large, deep jugular lymph nodes (Fig.7,8).
Occasionally, labelled macrophages were seen inside the
lumen of large, thin-walled subependymal brain vessels
suggesting emigration from brain by penetration of the vascular endothelium.

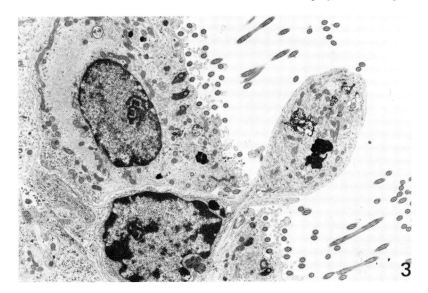

Fig. 3:
Intraependymally located microglia cell (lateral ventricle
bordering on the head of the caudate) with intraventricular
process involved in melanin uptake. 6 h after intraventricular 14C-5,6-DHT-melanin. x 6900

These observations indicate that four types of cells in
the CSF of the adult rat - which have previously been described as separate entities by several authors (Coates
1972; Bleier 1975; 1977; Ling 1978, for review, see
Oehmichen 1978) namely supraependymal, epiplexus, free subarachnoidal and perivascular cells of the CSF cisternes
behave as phagocytes upon challenge with an inert, particulate, synthetic melanin; these cells should be considered
as local variants of the same type of intrathecal resting
potential phagocyte, the morphology of which depends on regional environmental conditions. In addition, these cells
share properties with subependymal microglia-like cells
which are provided with intraventricular processes that remove melanin from the CSF by phagocytosis. Both the CSF-
resident and the subependymal phagocytes have the ability
to migrate into and across the brain parenchyma and to

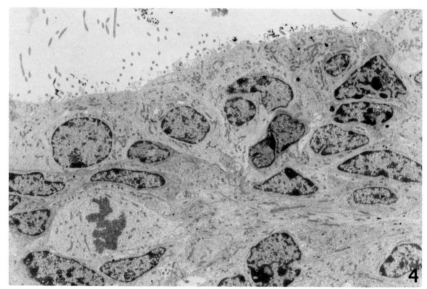

Fig. 4:
Head of the left lateral caudate nucleus, 2 days after 14-C-5,6-DHT-melanin injection. Note abundance of cells in the subependymal neuropil; one cell is undergoing mitotic division. x 3640

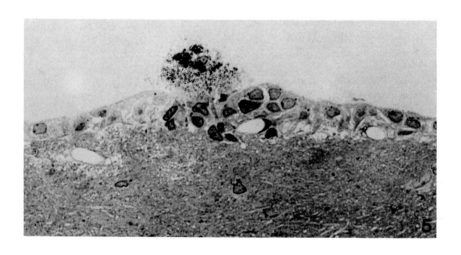

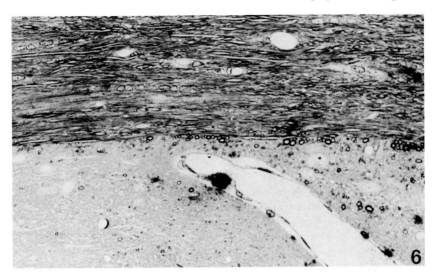

Fig. 6:

Light microscopic autoradiogram. Heavily labelled macrophage in the perivascular space of subcallosal brain vessel
(caudate nucleus) about to penetrate the endothelial lining.
8 days after 14C-5,6-DHT-melanin. x 500

settle in the perivascular space of brain vessels where
they eventually penetrate the endothelial lining to enter
the vascular lumen and thus the systemic circulation. Their
peripheral disposition remains to be clarified since we
have failed to locate labelled macrophages in the spleen,
lungs, kidneys or central portions of lymph nodes. That
melanin-loaded macrophages are cleared from the cisternal
CSF compartments via lymphatics or prelymphatics is strongly suggested by the appearance of labelled macrophages in
the marginal sinuses of the deep jugular lymph nodes by 4-
8 days after 14C-melanin injection thus confirming earlier

Fig. 5:
Light microscopic autoradiogram. Note grain clusters super-
imposed to a group of aggregated supraependymal cells and
grains concentrated over a macrophage perikaryon in the
perivascular space of subependymally located blood vessel.
4 days after 14C-5,6-DHT melanin. x 350

findings by Oehmichen (1978).

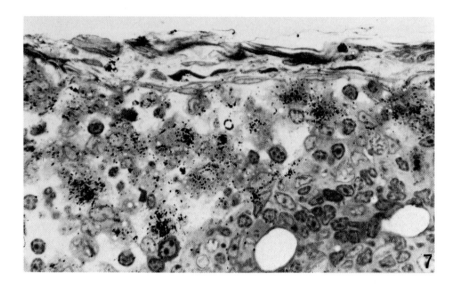

Fig.7:
Marginal sinus spaces of jugular lymph node,8 days after
14C-5,6-DHT-melanin. Note silver grain clusters over macro-
phage-like cells as identified in the consecutive electron-
micrograph (Fig. 8). x 560

Finally, it may be asked whether the present findings have
any bearing on the concept of the "graded respone on the
part of several, different sources of phagocytes" (Vaughn
and Pease 1970). In as much as the defined phagocytic stimulus applied (a particulate polymer resembling the biopo-
lymer melanin) provokes a uniform reaction of a homogeneous
system of CSF residing and subependymal phagocytes without
significant acute contribution of peripheral mononuclear
cells, our findings support the concept of a restricted
CNS phagocyte reaction in an experimental situation where
there is minimal alteration of the blood-brain-barrier.
In order to clarify the origin and replenishment of the
intrathecal phagocytes in more detail, studies combining
tritiated thymidine autoradiography with 14C-5,6-DHT-melanin
administration are in progress.

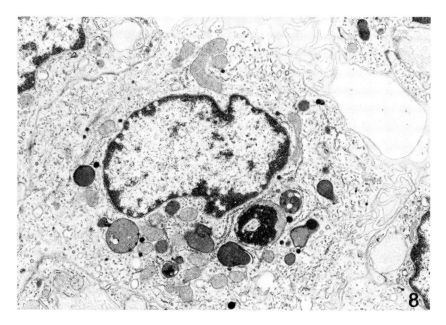

Fig. 8:
Detail from ultrathin section successive to the light micrograph depicted in Fig. 7. Macrophage with phagosomes one
of which stores masses of aggregated melanin particles.

REFERENCES

Bleier, R., Albrecht, R., Cruce, J.H.F.: Supraependymal
    cells of hypothalamic third ventricle: Identification
    as resident phagocytes of the brain. Science, 189: 299-
    301 (1975)

Bleier, R.: Ultrastructure of supraependymal cells and
    ependyma of hypothalamic third ventricle of mouse.
    J. Comp. Neur., 1974: 359-376 (1977)

Coates, P.W.: Supraependymal cells: light and transmission
    electron microscopy extends scanning electron microsco-
    pic demonstration. Brain Res., 57: 502-507 (1973)

Ling, E.A.: Ultrastructure and origin of epiplexus cells in the telencephalic choroid plexus of postnatal rats studied by intravenous injection of carbon particles. J.A. at., 479-492 (1978)

Moritz, F., Baumgarten, H.G., Schlossberger, H.G.: The disposition of intraventricularly injected. 14C-5,6-DHT-melanin in and possible routes of elimination from the rat CNS, an autoradiographic study. Cell Tiss. Res. (1980), in press

Oehmichen, M.: Mononuclear Phagocytes in the Central Nervous System, Springer-Verlag (1978) Berlin, Heidelberg, New York

Paterson, J.A., Privat, A., Ling, E.A., Leblond, C.P.: Investigation of glial cells in semithin sections. III. Transformation of subependymal cells into glia cells, as shown by radioautography after ^{3}H-thymidine injection into the lateral ventricle of the brain of young rats. J. Comp. Neur. 149, 83-102 (1973)

Vaughn, J.E., Pease, D.C.: Electron microscopic studies of Wallerian degeneration rat optic nerves. II. Astrocytes, oligodendrocytes and adventitial cells. J. Comp. Neurol. 140, 207-266 (1970)

MORPHOLOGICAL ASPECTS OF
INTERNEURONAL COMMUNICATION

Eleventh International Congress of Anatomy:
Glial and Neuronal Cell Biology, pages 199—215
© **1981 Alan R. Liss, Inc., 150 Fifth Avenue, New York, NY 10011**

QUANTITATION OF DEVELOPING AND ADULT SYNAPSES

G.Vrensen and L.Müller

Netherlands Ophthalmic Research Institute,
Dept.of Morphology,
P.O.Box 6411
1005 EK Amsterdam, (The Netherlands).

The pioneering work of Cajal and Sherrington, at the turn of the 19th century, on the structure and function of the brain has become the beginning of an era of most intensive brain research. Ever since, a wealth of information has accumulated regarding the electrophysiological, biochemical and morphological aspects of the brain. For many brain regions the basic circuitry and the main afferents and efferents have been traced, (Creutzfeldt, 1978, Hubel and Wiesel, 1979, Szentagothai, 1978, Nauta and Feirtag, 1979). The basic electrophysiological and molecular processes operating during synaptic transmission are largely understood and the intrinsic relation between synaptic function and synaptic fine structure is mainly elucidated, (McGeer, Eccles and McGeer, 1978, Kelly et al.1979, Pfenninger, 1978, Israel et al.,1979). Experimental and ontogenetic studies have shown that functional changes are accompanied with structural modifications at the neuronal and synaptic level, (Jacobson, 1978, Globus, 1975, Vrensen, 1978). Further progress towards a realistic understanding of the integrative functioning of neuronal networks awaits quantitative approaches of these basic processes. Quantitative morphological analysis of e.g. synaptic density, laminar and neuronal distribution of synaptic junctions, strength of the individual synapses and inhibitory vs. excitatory character of the terminals will significantly contribute to this realistic understanding. Especially the fact that quantitative ultrastructural studies provide us with detailed and topographically well-defined information makes this approach a favorable one. The recent introduction of a reliable Golgi-EM technique (Fairén et al. 1977) giving both adequate information on the Golgi architec-

SYNAPTIC ORGANIZATION

	Quantitation in:
● Synaptic Density	OsO$_4$, EPTA, BiUL, etc. Golgi (Spines) Preparations
● Laminar Distribution	ibid
● Neuronal Distribution of Synapses	Reduced Golgi – EM HRP – EM Serial Sections
● Neuronal Distribution of Specific Synapses	Reduced Golgi – EM Autoradiography, HRP Degeneration
● Inhibitory vs. Excitory Synapses	OsO$_4$, OZI, Specific staining
● Synaptic Efficacy	

NEURONAL NETWORK

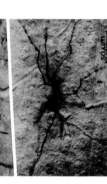

50 μm

HISTOLOGY

● Lamination

● Cell Types

● Extrinsic Afferents

  ● Specific, thalamic

  ● Callosal

  ● Intrahemispheric

● Intrinsic Connections
  interneurons

● Efferents

1

ture at the LM-level and detailed undisturbed information at the EM-level has greatly increased the potentialities of the quantitative approach of synaptic organization. Quantitative studies have significantly increased our knowledge on synaptic organization and it may be expected to contribute in future to a better understanding of a number of neurobiological questions as e.g.:

● The relation between synaptic maturation and onset of brain functioning, (Blakemore, 1975, Berry, 1974, Jacobson, 1978),

● The relation between intrinsic and environmental factors in brain maturation, (Changeux and Danchin, 1976, McGeer, Eccles and McGeer, 1978, Vrensen, 1978),

● The modifications and disturbances of the wiring diagram resulting from experimental manipulation as e.g. deprivation, selective or enriched input, lesions and undernutrition, (Barlow, 1975, Cotman and Nadler, 1978, Globus, 1975, Jones, 1976, Shoemaker and Bloom, 1977),

● The problem of neuronal recognition, (Appel, 1975, Hamburger, 1975, Pfenninger and Rees, 1976),

● The functional integration at the neuronal level, (Barrett, 1975, Koziol and Tuckwell, 1978),

● The brain mechanisms underlying learning and memory, (Cragg, 1974, Trubatch et al, 1977, Kandel, 1979, De Feudis and De Feudis, 1977, McGeer, Eccles and McGeer, 1978),

It will be clear that it is impossible, within the limited space and time available for this review, to discuss these items even superficially. Therefore we will restrict ourselves to a critical description of relevant quantitative synaptic parameters and to a short discussion on some aspects of synaptic ontogenesis.

Quantitative Synaptic Parameters

In Fig.1 the basic morphological aspects of a neuronal network are schematically summarized and the relevant quantitative parameters of synaptic organization are indicated. Overall density and laminar distribution of synaptic contacts have been investigated by numerous authors in many species and brain regions (for ref.see e.g. Vrensen, 1978 and Vrensen et al. 1977). This type of measurement is

straightforward and can be carried out on routinely treated
brain tissue (OsO4) using simple stereological procedures.
The use of the synapse-selective E-PTA (ethanolic-phospho-
tungstic acid) procedure, originally introduced by Bloom and
coworkers, (Bloom, 1972), greatly facilitates these measurements. Quantitation of overall synaptic density is most valuable and most often used for comparative studies on the effects of experimental manipulation e.g.malnutrition and visual deprivation (Barlow, 1975, Cotman and Nadler, 1978,
Globus, 1975, Jones, 1976, Shoemaker and Bloom, 1977, Vrensen, 1978). On account of these simple measurements the number of synaptic contacts per neuron can be calculated (e.g.
Cragg, 1975 and Vrensen et al. 1977).This may be a useful
value in theoretical considerations regarding the functional
integration of information at the neuronal level. However,
except for some specific brain regions, where only one or a
few cell types are present (see e.g.Koziol and Tuckwell,
1978), the disadvantage of the overall estimate of synaptic
density is that it necessarily neglects the variations among
cell types and the differences between cells of the same type.
      The counting of dendritic spines in Golgi-specimen is
a much more sophisticated method to study the cell specific
synaptic organization and has been used extensively for the
same type of experimental investigations as mentioned above,
(see e.g.Valverde, 1971, Greenough et al. 1975). However,
spine counting has its own disadvantages. Spines form only
part (small?) of the synaptic input to a restricted number
of spiny cell types, and spines have a specific electrophysiological function (Peters et al., 1976). As recently pointed out by Feldman and Peters (1979) counting of spines visible at the LM-level greatly underestimates the true number of spines, because the diameter of the dendritic shaft
and the size and length of the spines influence the countings.
The authors present a geometrically based method which
enables an estimate of spine density with an accuracy of
better than 10%. Freire (1978) recently reinvestigated the
effects of dark rearing on dendritic spines in layer IV of
the mouse visual cortex by means of quantitative EM. In
contrast with the original observation of Valverde (1971)
no reduction in dendritic spines was deduced, which is in
agreement with the observations of Vrensen and De Groot(1974)
in rabbits. A significant and remarkable reduction in the
mean size of the spines after dark rearing may explain this
apparent contradiction between spine density at the LM and
EM-level, because many of the reduced spines will be smaller
than the resolution limit of the LM.

Some 10 years ago the study of Golgi-impregnated neurons at the EM-level has been proposed as a most potential method to unravel the detailed synaptic organization of neurons and neuronal networks, (Blackstad, 1970). Due to technical problems, mainly concerning the adequate preservation and visualization of both the pre-and postsynaptic elements, this method has become operative only a few years ago, by the introduction of a reliable method by Fairén et al. (1977). The replacement of silver by gold in Golgi-impregnated brain tissue and the subsequent removal of the excess of silver fullfills the requirements for optimal EM-visualization. The method has already been used in a number of interesting descriptive papers. Although the quantitative potentialities of the Golgi-EM method and the comparable HRP-EM and specific dyes-EM methods are evident, only few papers have appeared using these methods (White and Rock, 1979). In our laboratory Meek (1980) has recently finished a study on the quantitative aspects of synaptic organization of the optic tectum of the goldfish, using the Golgi EM technique. Simple measuremnts reveal detailed information on the synaptic density of different cell types, the distribution of the contacts along the distinct components of the cell and the size of the contacts. The variation in number of synaptic contacts between different cell types and between neurons of the same type have become available. Some interesting general aspects of the synaptic organization can be inferred:

- the cellular distribution of synaptic contacts and the overall number per cell are rather specific for each cell type suggesting that synaptic density and distribution are determined postsynaptically by the target cells,
- the size of the synaptic contacts is rather specific for each lamina suggesting that the afferents establish contacts with a characteristic size.

Whether these inferences are restricted to the tectum or have a more general validity for all laminated brain regions must be further investigated. In the optic tectum the retinal afferents have characteristic fine structural features. So it was possible to approximate the number of retinal terminals on the different cell types and to estimate the relative contribution on the terminals to the total synaptic input. Combination of the Golgi-EM method with radioactive or HRP labelling of specific afferents will enable a further analysis of the synaptic organization along this line.

The common observation of spheroid and flat or pleo-

morphic vesicles of different size in the mammalian central
nervous system and the conjecture of Uchizono (1965) that
the presence of spheroid and flat vesicles reflect the excitatory and inhibitory character of the terminals respectively seem to make the analysis of these two types of terminals straightforward. However, Valdivia (1971) and Paula-
Barbosa (1975) have shown that the shape of the vesicles
strongly depends on some factors of the primary solution
used for fixation. Moreover, at present many (putative)
transmitters are known to operate so that a simple distinction between two shapes does not seem to be adequate. More
sophisticated methods are wanted to make a relevant distinction between different types of terminals as e.g.specific
histochemical staining and specific radioactive labelling
(Bloom, 1970).

The correlation between structure and function, a general objective of molecular biological research, seems to
be firmly established for the synapse. The pioneering studies of Palade, Palay, Gray, Bloom, Akert, Eccles, Katz,
Whittaker and many others have prompted the "vesicle hypothesis" as an explanation for transmitter release; the basic
phenomenon of synaptic transmission, (for a recent excellent review see Kelly et al., 1979). Recently an alternative: the "operator hypothesis", has been proposed by Israel
et al., (1979). The basic assumptions for relevant quantitative morphological research in this field are that there
exist an intrinsic relation between functional aspects of
the process of transmission and fine structural components
of the synaptic terminal and that functional changes are
accompanied with structural changes. A direct correlation
between transmitter release and synaptic vesicles and the
involvement of the presynaptic membrane and its specialization in this process is strongly suggested by the work of
Heuser and coworkers (1979) and Ceccarelli and Hurlbut,
(1975), at least for the neuromuscular junctions. The work
of Akert and coworkers (1975) has made it plausible that
identical processes are operative in the central nervous
system. Changes in number of synaptic vesicles in the cerebral cortex due to sensory input alterations (Garey and Pettigrew, 1974, Vrensen and De Groot, 1974 and Fehér et al.,
1972) seem to confirm the quantitative correlation between
synaptic vesicles and synaptic functioning for the central
nervous system. Some quantitative electrophysiological aspects of synaptic efficacy have been discussed by Kuno
(1974) and Martin, (1977). These authors conjecture that the
synaptic efficacy is mainly determined by presynaptic factors especially the mean quantum content and that modifica-

SYNAPTIC EFFICACY

$E = a.F.E_1$
Amplitude of EPSP

(:) Number of Afferents
a.F (:) Topography of Afferents
(:) Inhibitory vs. Excitatory

$E_1 = I_1.R.m$
Mean Amplitude of EPSP
evoked by single Afferents

I_1 Synaptic Current
R Input Resistance

m
Mean Quantum Content
(:) Amount of Transmitter
(:) Number of Release Sites
(:) Calcium Channels

(:) Number of Vesicles
(:) Number of Dense Projections
Kuno [1974]

Other Relevant Parameters

- Intercleft Space
- Intercleft Line
- Postsynaptic Band
- Mitochondria
- Spine Apparatus

- Size of Pre- and Postsynaptic Terminal
- Shape of the Active Zone
- annulate / horseshoe - shaped
- curvature

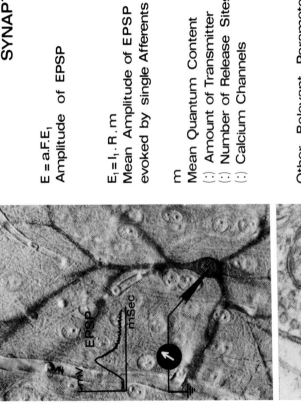

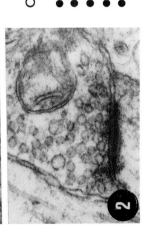

tions of synaptic strength are related to variations in the
quantum content. These basic aspects of synaptic efficacy
are summarized in Fig.2 and the emerging morphological
counterparts are indicated. Quantitation of synaptic vesicles is simple and can be performed on routinely treated
brain tissue. The use of the OZI-procedure (osmic-zinc iodi-
de), introduced by Akert and Sandri (1968) facilitates the
countings. Release sites and Ca^{++}-channels can be visualized
and counted in freeze-etch specimen (see Heuser and coworkers, 1979, and Akert et al. 1972). Recent investigations in
our laboratory, (Vrensen et al, 1980) suggest that release
sites and probably Ca^{++}-channels are complementary to the
dense projections as seen in the E-PTA specimen. The visualization of synaptic contacts, in full *en face* view, in semithin E-PTA sections enables a systematic study of the dense
projections and consequently of the alterations due to experimental manipulations (Vrensen, 1980). Besides the parameters directly involved in transmitter release, numerous
other morphological parameters may reflect changes in synaptic transmission. Diffusion and breakdown of the transmitter
may be related to the intercleft space and intercleft line.
The postsynaptic binding of the transmitter depends on the
receptors in the postsynaptic membrane and band. Moreover,
the size of the pre-and postsynaptic terminals, the presence
of mitochondria, spine apparatus etc. may reflect the general
metabolic integrity of the synapse. Recent observations of
Greenough et al. (1978), Vrensen et al., (1980) and Dyson
and Jones, (1980) have shown that the shape of the active
zones is subject to variations during ontogenesis and as a
result of experimental modification of the environment.
It is impossible, within the scope of this review, to summarize the numerous papers dealing with this aspect of synaptic quantitation. We like to conclude this paragraph with
two critical remarks. Fine structural quantitation has the
obvious advantage over biochemical studies that it can be
carried out on very specific parts of the brain and can be
restricted to specific synaptic contacts impinging on specific cell types. Coincidence of electrophysiological, behavioral and structural alterations does not necessarily imply
causal relation. Careful interdisciplinary approaches are
often required to proof causality.

Quantitation of Developing Synapses

    An intriguing aspect of brain development is the rela-
tion between intrinsic and environmental factors as determi-

nants of the structure and function of the mature brain.
Recent evidence indicates that intrinsic and environmental
factors differentially govern the two distinct aspects of
synaptic organization *viz.* the circuitry and the functioning
of the connections. Therefore it seems meaningful to discuss these aspects separately.

Synaptogenesis has been studied extensively in the cerebral cortex of vertebrates, (for ref. see Vrensen et al.,
1977, Dyson and Jones, 1980). Investigations in other brain
regions are rather fragmentary and do not allow general conclusions. Quantitative studies on synapse formation especially in the visual cortex show that the synaptogenic period
can be divided in two phases:
1. a slow phase starting prior to birth, levelling at about
   5-10 per cent of the adult level and persisting during
   the first postnatal week. Most investigators agree that
   the synapses at this stage are rather immature, have few
   synaptic vesicles and relatively undifferentiated synaptic contact zones. As pointed out by Kristt, (1978) the
   early synapses are concentrated at specific cortical
   depths which correspond to regions where the most-mature
   neuronal elements are found. The postnatal part of this
   period is characterized by a rapid development of the laminar organization and increase in thickness reaching adult
   levels at the end of the 1st postnatal week.
2. a rapid phase, starting at the turn of the 1st or half-
   way the 2nd week, characterized by an exponential increase in synaptic density and persisting up to the end
   of the 3rd or 4th postnatal week. At this time synaptic
   density has reached 90-120 per cent of the adult level.
   The onset of this exponential growth phase coincides with
   eye opening. This period is also characterized by a dramatic increase of neuronal size and elaboration of the
   dendritic pattern which reach maturity at the end of the
   3rd postnatal week, (Parnavelas and Uylings, 1980, Salas
   et al., 1974, Schierhorn, 1977).
The coincidence of eye opening and rapid synaptogenesis in
the visual cortex is rather suggestive with respect to the influence of visual input on the maturation of this brain region.
However, the correlation suggested by this coincidence is
only apparent. Quantitative studies have shown that a similar
sequence of synaptogenesis exists in other non-visual areas.
Moreover, if visual input would be an important trigger for
the development of the circuitry of the visual cortex some
prerequisites must be fulfilled:

1. the presence of specific functional and morphological afferent pathways; for the visual cortex the retino-genicu-
   late-cortical pathway.
2. the relay of relevant visual information from the eye to
   the visual cortex depends on maturation of the image-for-
   ming media and complete or partial maturation of the synaptic pattern of retina and geniculate nucleus,
3. visual deprivation will affect the development of the cortical circuitry.

Lund and Bunt, (1976) and Höllander et al., (1979) have shown
that in rabbits and rats the main afferents and efferents of
the visual cortex are present at birth. Recent investigations
in our laboratory have shown that transport of radioactive
proline and fucose to the geniculate and colliculus starts
abruptly at about postnatal day 7 but is absent at day 3. The
quantitative studies of Fisher, (1979) and Cragg, (1975) have
shown that the main synaptogenic period in the retina and lateral geniculate nucleus largely parallels the synaptogenesis
in the visual cortex. This means that it is not detailed visual
information which governs the maturation of cortical circuitry.
The most relevant assumption that can be made is that the few
synaptic contacts present in these early stages relay some
information about the presence or absence of light in the environment. Numerous studies have dealt with the effects of deprivation on the organization of the visual cortex. The present evidence indicates that input restriction does not affect
the mature synaptic organization of the visual cortex. Retardation of the development of e.g. specific synaptic connections as suggested by the spine countings on layer V pyramids
by Valverde (1971) cannot be excluded, although the reinvestigation by Freire, (1978) of this material makes this conclusion questionable (see previous paragraph on synaptic density in this paper). Whether deprivation affects the neuronal
distribution of the connections, as is suggested by the alterations in tuning of the cortical neurons after monocular deprivation (cf.e.g. Hubel and Wiesel, 1979), has not been investigated up till now. Golgi-EM studies seem to be most suitable
for this. However, studies on the laminar distribution of synapses in control and dark reared animals do not show gross
changes. Moreover, visual evoked potentials after long term
dark rearing or monocular deprivation exhibit similar deflec-
tions as control animals but with reduced amplitude (Kobayashi and Van Hof, 1972, Singer, 1978). After an initial adaptation period, dark reared and monocular deprived rabbits and
cats show a remarkable ability for visual discrimination learning largely resembling that of control animals (Van Hof and

Kobayashi, 1972 and Van Hof-Van Duin, 1976). Further relevant
indications regarding the basic question of sensory input and
cortical development are given by the study of synaptogenesis
in the quinea pig which is nearly finished at birth in this
prenatal brain developer (Jones et al.,1974) and by studies
of synaptogenesis in tissue culture which show that the formation of synapses in vitro can be compared with the in vivo
sequence even with respect to timing (Burry and Lasher, 1978,
Romijn, personal communication, Pfenninger and Rees, 1976),

- The conclusion emerging from present studies on synaptogenesis is that the circuitry of a brain region is mainly determined by intrinsic (genetic and epigenetic) factors. How these genetic factors operate and control the
  growth of neurons and synapses is not fully understood
  and cannot be discussed in this review.

A consequence of the previous conclusion, that the development of the circuitry is mainly determined by intrinsic
factors, is that the plasticity of the nervous system, so evident from electrophysiological and behavioral studies cannot
be ascribed to a steady reorganization of the synaptic connections and that some other mechanism must be at work. A
plausible explanation for such a mechanism is the functional
adaptation of the existing, pre-wired connections. Changes in
the efficacy of the majority of synaptic connections after
dark rearing or differential variations in the efficacy of
ipsi-and contralateral connections after monocular deprivation can basically explain the electrophysiological and
behavioral changes. Arguments in favor of this view have been
found in studies on the normal and disturbed development of
synapses. Investigations by Dyson and Jones, (1976, 1980),
Armstrong and Johnson (1970), De Groot and Vrensen (1978),
Jones and Cullen (1979) , Bloom (1972), Greenough et al. (1978),
Jones et al. (1974), Adinolfi (1972), Vrensen et al. (1977)
have shown that the synaptic active zones and their paramembranous densities, the size of the presynaptic terminals, the
synaptic vesicles, the curvature of the synaptic contacts and
the frequency of annulate and horseshoe-shaped synaptic contacts, gradually increase during the postnatal period and is
continuing after completion of synaptic density. This indicates that these parameters which are considered as morphological indications of synaptic functioning mature during the
period of detailed visual input and thus may be subject to
functional verification. The studies of Garey and Pettigrew
(1974) and Vrensen and De Groot (1974, 1975) showing that
dark rearing and monocular deprivation give rise to signifi-

cant diminution of synaptic vesicles confirm this view. A recent investigation in our laboratory (Müller and Vrensen, 1980) of the development of the synaptic grid has shown that dark rearing seriously affects the maturation of dense projections, indicating and impairment of the vesicle releasing ability of the synapses.

● A tentative conclusion of these studies on the development of synaptic fine structure is that functional validation and/or consolidation of synaptic efficacy is most likely an important factor in regulating neuronal plasticity.

From the quantitative studies on synaptogenesis, briefly summarized here, the following tentative conjecture can be inferred:

● The structural, histological and electron microscopic organization of cortical neuronal networks is mainly regulated by intrinsic factors and is largely independent of sensory input. Functional validation and/or consolidation of the pre-wired connections is affected by environmental factors and may be an important aspect of neuronal plasticity.

This conjecture based on morphological observations is in good agreement with the conjecture of Singer (1978) based on electrophysiological observations that "experience dependent changes in neuronal circuitry are based on a selection process among pre-existing excitatory connections".

Selected References

Adinolfi AM (1972). The organization of paramembranous densities during postnatal maturation of synaptic junctions in the cerebral cortex. Experimental Neurology 34:383.

Akert K, Peper K (1975). Ultrastructure of chemical synapses: A comparison between presynaptic membrane complexes of the motor end plate and the synaptic junction in the central nervous system. In Santini M (ed): "Golgi Centennial Symposium", New York: Raven Press, p 521.

Akert K, Sandri C (1968). An electron microscope study of zinc-iodide-osmium impregnation of neurons. I Staining of synaptic vesicles at cholinergic junctions. Brain Research 7:286.

Akert K, Sandri C (1975). Significance of the Maillet method for cytochemical studies of synapses. In Santini M (ed): "Golgi Centennial Symposium", New York: Raven Press, p 387.

Akert K, Pfenninger K, Sandri C, Moor H (1972). Freeze etch-

ing and cytochemistry of vesicles and membrane complex-
es in synapses of the central nervous system. In Pappas
GD, Purpura DP (eds): "Structure and Function of Synapses",
New York: Raven Press, p 67.

Appel SH (1975). Neuronal recognition and synaptogenesis.
Experimental Neurology 48:52.

Armstrong-James M, Johnson R (1970). Quantitative studies
of postnatal changes in synapses in rat superficial motor
cerebral cortex. An electron microscopical study. Z Zellforsch 110:559.

Barlow HB (1975). Visual experience and cortical development. Nature 258:199.

Barrett NJ (1975). Motoneuron dendrites: Role in synaptic
integration. Fed.Proc 34:1398.

Berry M (1974). Development of the cerebral neocortex of
the rat. In Gottlieb G (ed): "Aspects of Neurogenesis",
New York: Academic Press, p 8.

Blackstad TW (1970). Electron microscopy of Golgi prepara-
tions for the study of neuronal relations. In Nauta WJH,
Ebbeson SOE (eds):"Contemporary Research Methods in
Neuroanatomy", Heidelberg: Springer Verlag, p 186.

Blakemore C (1975). Development of functional connections in
the mammalian visual system. In Brazier MAB (ed): "Growth
and Development of the Brain", New York: Raven Press,p
157.

Bloom FE (1970). Correlating structure and function of synaptic ultrastructure. In Schmitt FO (ed):"The Neurosciences", New York: The Rockefeller University Press, p 729.

Bloom FE (1972). The formation of synaptic junctions in
developing rat brain. In Pappas GD, Purpura DP (eds):
"Structure and Function of Synapses", New York: Raven
Press, p 101.

Burry RW, Lasher RS (1978). A quantitative electron microscopic study of synapse formation in dispersed cell cultures of rat cerebellum stained either by Os-Ul or by
E-PTA. Brain Research 147:1.

Ceccarelli B, Hurlbut WP (1976). Transmitter release and
the vesicle hypothesis. In Santini M (ed): "Golgi Centennial Symposium", New York: Raven Press, p 529.

Changeux JP, Danchin A (1975). Selective stabilisation of
developing synapses as a mechanism for the specification
of neuronal networks. Nature 264:705.

Cotman CW, Nadler JV (1978). Reactive synaptogenesis in the
hippocampus. In Cotman CW (ed): "Neuronal Plasticity",
New York: Raven Press, p 227.

Cragg BG (1974). Plasticity of synapses. Br Med Bull 30:141.

Cragg BG (1975). The development of synapses in kitten vi-
vual cortex during visual deprivation. Experimental Neurology 46:445.

Cragg BG (1975). The development of synapses in the visual
system of the cat. J Comp Neurol 160:147.

Creutzfeldt OD (1978). The neocortical link:Thoughts on
the generality of structure and function of the neocortex.
In Brazier MAB, Petsche H (eds): "Architectonics of the
Cerebral Cortex", New York: Raven Press, p 357.

De Feudis FV, De Feudis PAF (1977). "Elements of the Behavioral Code", London: Academic Press.

Dyson SE, Jones DG (1976). Some effects of undernutrition
on synaptic development: a quantitative ultrastructural
study. Brain Research 114:365.

Dyson SE. Jones, DG (1980). Quantitation of terminal parameters and their interrelationships in maturing central
synapses: a perspective for experimental studies. Brain
Research 183:43.

Fairén A, Peters A, Saldanha J (1977). A new procedure for
examining Golgi-impregnated neurons by light and electron
microscopy. J Neurocyt 6:311.

Fehér O, Joó F, Halasz N (1972). Effect of stimulation on
the number of synaptic vesicles in nerve fibers and terminals of the cerebral cortex in the cat. Brain Research
47:37.

Feldman ML, Peters A (1979). A technique for estimating total
spine numbers on Golgi-impregnated dendrites, J Comp Neurol
188:527.

Fisher LJ (1979). Development of retinal synaptic arrays in
the inner plexiform layer of dark-reared mice. J Embryol
and Exp Morphology 54:219.

Freire M (1978). Effects of dark rearing on dendritic spines
in layer IV of the mouse visual cortex. A quantitative
electron microscopical study. J Anat 126:193.

Garey LJ, Pettigrew JD (1974). Ultrastructural changes in
kitten visual cortex after environmental modification.
Brain Research 66:165.

Globus A (1975). Brain morphology as a function of presynaptic morphology and activity. In Riesen AH (ed): "The Developmental Neurophysiology of Sensory Deprivation", New York:
Academic Press, p 9.

Greenough WT (1976). Enduring brain effects of differential
experience and training. In Rosenzweig MR, Bennett EL (eds):
"Neural Mechanisms of Learning and Memory", Cambridge:
MIT Press, p 255.

Greenough WT, West RW, De Voogd TJ (1978). Subsynaptic plate perforations: changes with age and experience in the rat. Science 202:1096.

Hamburger V (1975). Changing concepts in developmental neurobiology. Persp Biol Med 18:162.

Heuser JE, Reese TS, Dennis MJ, Jan Y, Jan L, Evans L (1979). Synaptic vesicle exocytosis captured by quick freezing and correlated with quantal transmitter release. J Cell Biol 81:275.

Holländer H, Tietze J, Distel H (1979). An autoradiographic study of the subcortical projections of the rabbit striate cortex in the adult and during postnatal development. J Comp Neurol 184:783.

Hubel DH, Wiesel TN (1979). Brain mechanisms of vision. Scientific American 241:150.

Israel M, Dunant Y, Manaranche R (1979). The present status of the vesicular hypothesis. Progress Neurobiology 13:237.

Jacobson M (1978), "Developmental Neurobiology". New York: Plenum Press, p 181.

Jones DG (1976). The vulnerability of the brain to undernutrition. Sci Prog Oxf 63:483.

Jones DG, Cullen AM (1979). A quantitative investigation of some presynaptic terminal parameters during synaptogenesis. Experimental Neurology 64:245.

Jones DG, Dittmer MM, Reading LC (1974). Synaptogenesis in guinea-pig cerebral cortex: A glutaraldehyde PTA study. Brain Research 70:245.

Kandel ER (1979). Small systems of neurons. Scientific American 241:66.

Kelly RB, Deutsch JW, Carlson SS, Wagner JA (1979). Biochemistry of neurotransmitter release. Ann Rev Neurosci 2:399.

Kobayashi K, Van Hof MW (1972). Visual evoked responses in rabbits deprived of light for seven months after birth. Acta Soc Ophthalm Jap 76(5):257.

Koziol JA, Tuckwell HC (1978). Analysis and estimation of synaptic densities and their spatial variation on the motoneuron surface. Brain Research 150:617.

Kristt DA (1978). Neuronal differentiation of somatosensory cortex of the rat. I Relationship to synaptogenesis in the first postnatal week. Brain Research 150:467.

Kuno M (1974). Factors in efficacy of central synapses. In Bennett MVL (ed): "Synapic Transmission and Neuronal Interaction", New York: Raven Press, p 79.

Lund RD, Bunt AH (1976). Prenatal development of central optic pathways in albino rats. J Comp Neurol 165:247.

Martin AR, (1977). Junctional transmission. II Presynaptic mechanisms. In Brookhart JM, Mountcastle VB, Kandel ER,

Geiger SR (eds): "Handbook of Physiology, The Nervous System", vol I/1, Bethesda: Amer Physiol Soc, p 329.

McGeer PL, Eccles JC (1978). "Molecular Neurobiology of the
mammalian Brain". New York: Plenum Press.

Meek J (1980). A Golgi-electron microscopic study of goldfish optic tectum. II Quantitative aspects of synaptic
organization. J Comp Neurol. Submitted.

Nauta WJH, Feirtag M (1979). The organization of the brain.
Scientific American 241:88.

Parnavelas JG, Uylings HBM (1980). The growth of non-pyramidal neurons in the visual cortex of the rat: A morphome-
tric study. Brain Research 199: In Press.

Paula-Barbosa M (1975). The duration of aldehyde fixation
as a "flattening factor" of synaptic vesicles. Cell Tiss
Res 164:63.

Peters A, Palay SL, Webster H de F (1976). "The Fine Structure of the Nervous System: The Neurons and Supporting
Cells". Philadelphia: Saunders, Ch V.

Pfenninger KH (1978). Organization of neuronal membranes.
Ann Rev Neurosci 1:445.

Pfenninger KH, Rees RP (1976). From the growth cone to the
synapse. In Barondes SH (ed): "Neuronal Recognition",
London: Chapman and Hall, p 131.

Salas M, Diaz S, Nieto A (1974). Effects of neonatal food
deprivation on cortical spines and dendritic development
of the rat. Brain Research 73:139.

Schierhorn H (1977). Postnatale Entwicklung der Corticalen
Pyramidenzellen von Ratte und Katze. Verh Anat Ges 71:157.

Shoemaker WJ, Bloom FE (1977). Effect of undernutrition on
brain morphology. In Wurtman RJ, Wurtman JJ (eds): "Nutrition and the Brain", New York: Raven Press, p 148.

Singer W (1978). Neuronal mechanisms in experience dependent
modification of the visual cortex function. Progr Brain
Research 48:457.

Szentágothai J (1978). Specificity versus (quasi-) random-
ness in cortical connectivity. In Brazier MAB, Petsche H
(eds): "Architectonics of the Cerebral Cortex", New York:
Raven Press, p 77.

Trubatch J, Loud AV, Van Harreveld A (1977), Quantitative
stereological evaluation of KCL-induced ultrastructural
changes in frog brain. Neuroscience 2:963.

Uchizono K (1965). Characteristics of excitatory and inhibitory synapses in the central nervous system of the cat.
Nature 207:642.

Valdivia O (1971). Methods of fixation and the morphology
of synaptic vesicles. J Comp Neurol 142:257.

Valverde F (1971). Rate and extent of recovery from dark
    rearing in the visual cortex of the mouse. Brain Research
    33:1.
Van Hof-van Duin J (1976). Early and permanent effects of
    monocular deprivation on pattern discrimination and vi-
    suomotor behavior in cats. Brain Research 111:261.
Van Hof MW, Kobayashi K (1972). Pattern discrimination in
    rabbits deprived of light for 7 months after birth.
    Experimental Neurology 35:551.
Vrensen G (1978). Ontogenesis of the visual cortex of rab-
    bits and the effects of visual deprivation. In Corner MA,
    Baker RE, Van de Pol NE, Swaab DF, Uylings HBM (eds):
    "Maturation of the Nervous System, Progr Brain Res", Am-
    sterdam: Elsevier North-Holland Biomedical Press, p 231.
Vrensen G, De Groot D (1974). The effect of dark rearing
    and its recovery on synaptic terminals in the visual cor-
    tex of rabbits. A quantitative electron microscopic study.
    Brain Research 78:263.
Vrensen G, De Groot D (1975). The effect of monocular depri-
    vation on synaptic terminals in the visual cortex of rab-
    bits. A quantitative electron microscopic study. Brain
    Research 93:15.
Vrensen G, De Groot D, Nunes Cardozo J (1977). Postnatal
    development of neurons and synapses in the visual and
    motor cortex of rabbits. A quantitative light and electron
    microscopic study. Brain Res Bull 2:405.
Vrensen G, Nunes Cardozo J, Müller L, Van der Want J, (1980).
    The presynaptic grid. A new approach. Brain Research 184:
    23.
White EL, Rock MP (1979). Distribution of thalamic input to
    different dendrites of a spiny stellate cell in mouse
    sensorimotor cortex. Neurosci Letters 15:115.

Eleventh International Congress of Anatomy:
Glial and Neuronal Cell Biology, pages 217—227
© 1981 Alan R. Liss, Inc., 150 Fifth Avenue, New York, NY 10011

SYNAPTIC ULTRASTRUCTURE IN UNANESTHETIZED AND EXPERIMENTALLY
MODIFIED CEREBRAL CORTEX

D.G. Jones

Department of Anatomy and Human Biology,
University of Western Australia,
Nedlands, W.A. 6009, Australia.

Until the early 1970's few attempts had been made to
quantify synaptic ultrastructure, investigations having
been directed towards estimating synaptic density and, to
a lesser extent, synaptic connectivity. Useful as these
counts have proved, particularly in experimental investigations, they are limited in scope and fail to answer the
question of how synapses, as organizational units, undergo
modification during development and in response to various
experimental demands.

In an attempt to bridge this gap the ethanolic phosphotungstic acid (E-PTA) technique has been employed as a
means of quantifying synaptic development. The usefulness
of this technique stems from its ability to exploit the
orderliness of the paramembranous densities at synaptic junctions (Bloom, 1972; Jones and Brearley, 1972; Vrensen and
De Groot, 1973). Of these densities, emphasis has been laid
on the presynaptic vesicular grid (Akert *et al.*, 1969;
Vrensen *et al.*, 1980), the arrangement of individual dense
projections within the grid (Jones *et al.*, 1974; Burry and
Lasher, 1978), and the length of the postsynaptic thickening –
synaptic length (Vrensen and De Groot, 1973; Jones, 1978).

Attempts at quantifying presynaptic terminal parameters
have used aldehyde-osmium material. Parameters of interest
are shown in Fig. 1. Of these, greatest attention has been
paid to the number of vesicles per terminal (Armstong-James
and Johnson, 1970; Vrensen *et al.*, 1977; Jones and Cullen,
1979), and this has proved a reliable indicator of terminal
maturity. Additional parameters include the sectional area

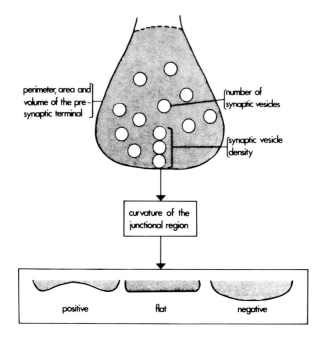

Fig. 1. Diagrammatic representation of a presynaptic terminal, with some of its commonly measured parameters.
The lower diagram indicates the different directions
of synaptic curvature.

and volume of the terminal (Armstrong-James and Johnson, 1970),
the curvature of its junctional region (Streit *et al.*, 1972;
Jones and Devon, 1978) and the frequency of intraterminal
profiles.

SYNAPTOGENESIS

When applied to analyses of synaptogenic events, junction parameters provide valuable information about the
changing status of developing synaptic junctions. They can
also be employed as a means of assessing junction maturity
(Dyson and Jones, 1976), by relying upon the appearance of
synaptic junctions as whole units. They do not however,
provide much information about the organization of the term-

inal itself. In order to do this, emphasis on the vesicles and other terminal profiles is required.

During synaptogenesis there is a dramatic increase in the number of synaptic vesicles per unit area within terminals (Armstrong-James and Johnson, 1970). This numerical increase is not accompanied by an equivalent size increase. Rather, vesicle size either remains constant (Burry and Lasher, 1978) or decreases (Larramendi *et al.*, 1967; Jones and Cullen, 1979) during synaptogenesis.

Presynaptic terminal size is variously expressed as volume, area and perimeter, and the results to date are conflicting. There appears to be fluctuation in terminal size during the developmental period with an overall decrease in size by the end of this period (Armstrong-James and Johnson, 1970; Jones and Cullen, 1979). During early adult life there is either an increase in size or a stabilization. By contrast, another study (Dyson and Jones, 1980) revealed a gradual enlargement of the terminals with maturation (15-224 days) in rat cerebral cortex. These differences may be attributable, in part, to the different criteria used for delineation of the terminal boundaries, while an additional contributing factor may be regional variation either within the cortex or even between cortical layers. It is even possible that the precise ways in which synaptic contacts within a particular synaptic population are constructed varies under different environmental pressures.

Synaptic curvatures can be subdivided into various curvature classes, ranging from flat junctions (class A) to highly curved ones (class M) in both the negative and positive directions (Fig. 1). The intermediate classes (B-L) represent junctions of increasing curvature. At day 15 in rat cerebral cortex curvatures extend relatively uniformly within both the negative and positive ranges of the scale, the overall distribution being bimodal (Dyson and Jones, 1980; Fig. 2). With increasing age the frequency of relatively flat junctions increases and there is a shift in the entire population towards a flatter type of junction. This is particularly marked at day 224 when the entire population appears to be normally distributed and the negative/positive dichotomy is masked (Dyson and Jones, 1980). With development, there is also a change in the way in which the entire population is distributed; a larger proportion of the population is negative rather than positive at the younger ages,

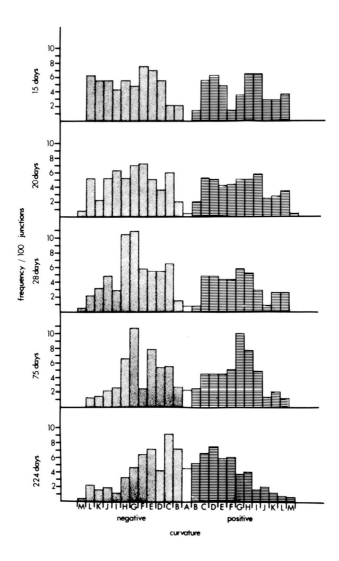

Fig. 2   The frequency distribution of synaptic curvature
classes at various developmental ages in rat cerebral cortex.   Class A junctions are flat ones;
classes B-M represent junctions of increasing curvature (from Dyson and Jones, 1980).

and more or less equivalent at the older ages (Fig. 2).

By relating individual parameters to each other, flat junctions emerge as the longest and the most highly curved junctions as the shortest. Further, the terminal areas of positive junctions are greater than those of negative ones (Dyson and Jones, 1980; Jones and Devon, 1980). This increasing diversity of parameters is leading to the formulation of a model of the developing cortical synapse.

UNANESTHETIZED SYNAPSES

The potential of synaptic quantitation is also being realized in studies of unanesthetized synaptic ultrastructure. In adult synapses increasing doses of pentobarbitone are accompanied by changes in synaptic curvature (Jones and Devon, 1977, 1978). There is a marked increase in curvature negativity over a 0-80 mg/kg dose range and a decrease in negativity at higher dose levels. The increase in curvature negativity is accompanied by an increase in synaptic length and dense projection numbers, with a consonant increase in the perimeter and area of the presynaptic terminal. Reversal of the negativity trend at higher dose levels is paralleled by reversal of these accompanying trends. Additionally, 'excess' intraterminal membrane is found in unanesthetized and in the 160-400 mg/kg material (Jones and Devon, 1978). This excess intraterminal membrane intermingles with synaptic vesicles and is in the form of double-membrane profiles, vacuoles, cisternae, tubular profiles and coated vesicles. Another feature is the increased frequency with which exocytotic sites occur at the presynaptic membrane in the unanesthetized material: 80% of terminals in cannulated material and 61% in stunned material (Devon and Jones, 1979).

Studies from other laboratories have underscored these findings. Turner (1977), for instance, in a combined pentobarbitone-HRP study, noted that at a 40 mg/kg dose of pentobarbitone there is a significant decrease in the number of peroxidase-labelled vesicles in cortical synaptic terminals. He concluded that pentobarbitone exerts an inhibitory effect on vesicular membrane transport and synaptic vesicle turnover. Hajós *et al.* (1978), using rat cortical synaptosomes, found that pentobarbitone decreases the number of synaptic vesicles attached to the presynaptic membrane,

implicating once again the presynaptic terminal as one of
the foci of pentobarbitone action. Even more interesting
is the consistent involvement of the synaptic vesicles,
particularly their reformation, migration and exocytosis, in
the process. Membrane recycling appears to be partially
responsible for these pentobarbitone-induced changes at
synapses, and may account for the observed synaptic curvature
changes.

When the effects of pentobarbitone on the sequence of
synaptic developmental events are studied, pentobarbitone
appears to have little influence on synaptic organization
until 15 days postnatal in rat cerebral cortex. Subsequently,
however, striking divergences become evident. In particular,
the percentage of terminals displaying vesicle attachment
sites increases markedly from 21-75 days in the unanesthetized material, but decreases over the same period in the
anesthetized.

Synapses from young material are more negatively-curved
than those from 21- and 75-day material in the unanesthetized
state. A similar trend is not present in the anesthetized
material, in which the relative negativity of the synapses
remains throughout development (Fig. 3). Accompanying these
changes is an increase in perimeter of the unanesthetized
terminals between 21 and 75 days, but a decrease in anesthetized terminals.

Parameters of particular interest are the mean number of
vesicles per terminal and the density of the vesicles in the
vicinity of the presynaptic membrane. When these are compared
it is noticeable that, whereas both increase during development in the unanesthetized state, the mean vesicle density
decreases with increasing age in the anesthetized material.
Analysis of these parameters, therefore, reveals a disjunc-
tion between them and hence a modification to the distribution of the vesicles in adult terminals following the use of
pentobarbitone.

SYNAPTIC ULTRASTRUCTURE FOLLOWING MALNUTRITION

The maturity of synaptic junctions as structural units
appears to be undermined by malnutrition. Using the E-PTA
technique it has been demonstrated that rat brains malnourished during early postnatal development are characterized by a

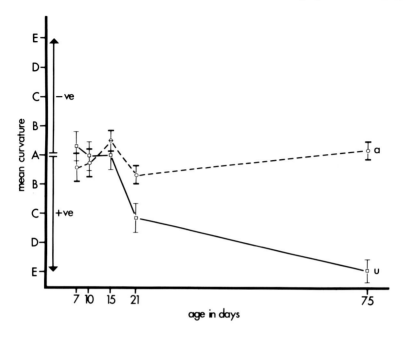

Fig. 3 Graphs of the mean values for synaptic curvature at
various ages during development in unanesthetized (u)
and anesthetized (a) rat cerebral cortex. Junctions
with curvature A are flat. The vertical lines represent standard errors of the mean.

shift towards the immature end of the synaptic continuum
(Dyson and Jones, 1976). This delayed synaptic development
can be detected by treating the junctional zone of synapses
as an integral unit.

The question, which now arises, is whether synaptic
parameters in aldehyde-osmium material are as helpful in
assessing synaptic maturity in a malnutrition model. Fig. 4
summarizes the overall synaptic parameter changes obtained
when control and protein-deficient rats at various ages from
15-224 days postnatal are compared. From this it can be seen
that all the parameters at 15 and 20 days are deficient in
the protein-deprived animals. All parameters, however, with
the exception of the area of the presynaptic terminal, are

either equivalent to or above the control values at 224 days.

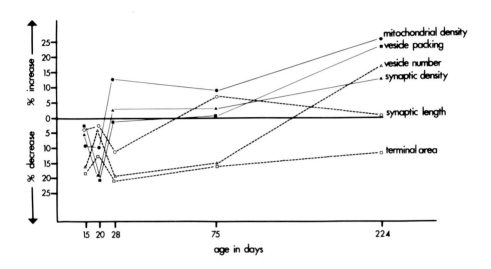

Fig. 4   Graphs depicting the percentage variation of quantitative synaptic parameters in protein-deprived
rats compared to controls. Variations in parameter
values from mean control values are expressed as
percentages of the control values.

When synaptic curvature trends in protein-deficient
animals are compared with those in control ones, it emerges
that at 15 days the deficit in positive junctions is more
pronounced than in control material. An approximate equivalence of negative and positive junctions is found in the
protein-deficient material at 20, 28 and 75 days, whereas
this equivalence occurs only at 75 and 224 days in the control junctions. At 224 days the proportion of positive
junctions is higher in the protein-deprived than in the control situation.

CONCLUSIONS

These quantitative approaches to synaptic ultrastructure have a potential for uncovering subtle functional variations. This has already proved of value in two ways. In unanesthetized investigations, they have provided a means of assessing different techniques for obtaining synapses in a near-functional state (Devon and Jones, 1979). They have also proved helpful in assessing synaptic maturity following malnutrition. The most useful synaptic parameters in these connections are: synaptic curvature, frequency of vesicle attachment sites, and vesicle packing density within terminals. While presynaptic terminal parameters are not as easy to interpret as those of the junctional zone, they may have more far-reaching implications as they appear to be pinpointing more discrete ultrastructural trends.

ACKNOWLEDGEMENTS

I should like to thank Mrs. Barbara Telfer for technical assistance. Mr. Richard Devon and Mrs. Susan Dyson were responsible for various facits of this study. Financial assistance was provided by TVW Telethon Foundation (Western Australia) and the Australian Research Grants Committee.

REFERENCES

Akert K, Moor H, Pfenninger K, Sandri K (1969). Contributions of new impregnation methods and freeze etching to the problems of synaptic fine structure. Prog Brain Res 31: 223.
Armstrong-James M, Johnson R (1970). Quantitative studies of postnatal changes in synapses in rat superficial motor cerebral cortex. An electron microscopical study. Z Zellforsch 110: 559.
Bloom FE (1972). The formation of synaptic junctions in developing rat brain. In Pappas GD, Purpura DP (eds): "Structure and Function of Synapses", New York: Raven Press, p 101.
Burry RW, Lasher RS (1978). A quantitative electron microscopic study of synapse formation in dispersed cell cultures of rat cerebellum stained either by Os-UL or by E-PTA. Brain Res 147: 1.

Devon RM, Jones DG (1979). Synaptic terminal parameters in unanaesthetized rat cerebral cortex. Cell Tissue Res 203: 189.

Dyson SE, Jones DG (1976). The morphological categorization of developing synaptic junctions. Cell Tissue Res 167: 363.

Dyson SE, Jones DG (1980). Quantitation of terminal parameters and their interrelationships in maturing central synapses: a perspective for experimental studies. Brain Res 183: 43.

Hajós, F, Csillag A, Kalman M (1978). The effect of pentobarbital, chlorohydrate, either and protoveratrine on the distribution of synaptic vesicles in rat cortical synaptosomes. Exp Brain Res 33: 91.

Jones DG (1978). "Some Current Concepts of Synaptic Organization". Berlin: Springer-Verlag.

Jones DG, Brearley RF (1972). Further studies on synaptic junctions. I and II. Z Zellforsch 125: 415.

Jones DG, Cullen AM (1979). A quantitative investigation of some presynaptic terminal parameters during synaptogenesis. Exp Neurol 64: 245.

Jones DG, Devon RM (1977). The influence of pentobarbitone on the distribution of membrane in cortical synapses. Neurosci Lett 6: 177

Jones DG, Devon RM (1978). An ultrastructural study into the effects of pentobarbitone on synaptic organization. Brain Res 147: 47.

Jones DG, Devon RM (1980). An analysis of the association between various synaptic parameters during cortical development. Cell Tissue Res, 208: 237.

Jones DG, Dittmer MM, Reading LC (1974). Synaptogenesis in guinea-pig cerebral cortex: a glutaraldehyde-PTA study. Brain Res 70: 245.

Larramendi LMH, Fickenscher L, Lemkey-Johnston N (1967). Synaptic vesicles of inhibitory and excitatory terminals in the cerebellum. Science 156: 967.

Streit P, Akert K, Sandri C, Livingston RB, Moor H (1972). Dynamic ultrastructure of presynaptic membranes at nerve terminals in the spinal cord of rats. Anesthetized and unanesthetized preparations compared. Brain Res 48: 11.

Turner PT (1977). Effect of pentobarbital on uptake of horseradish peroxidase by rabbit cortical synapses. Exp Neurol 54: 24.

Vrensen G, De Groot D (1973). Quantitative stereology of synapses: a critical investigation. Brain Res 58: 25.

Vrensen G, De Groot D, Nunes-Cardozo J (1977). Postnatal
    development of neurons and synapses in the visual and
    motor cortex of rabbits: a quantitative light and
    electron microscope study. Brain Res Bull 2: 405.
Vrensen G, Nunes-Cardozo J, Muller L, Van der Want J (1980)
    The presynaptic grid: a new approach. Brain Res 184: 23.

Eleventh International Congress of Anatomy:
Glial and Neuronal Cell Biology, pages 229—245
© 1981 Alan R. Liss, Inc., 150 Fifth Avenue, New York, NY 10011

PLASTICITY OF SYNAPTIC SIZE WITH CONSTANCY OF TOTAL SYNAPTIC
CONTACT AREA ON PURKINJE CELLS IN THE CEREBELLUM

D.E. Hillman and S. Chen

Department of Physiology and Biophysics

New York University Medical Center
550 First Avenue, NY   10016   USA

INTRODUCTION

A search for factors that control organization of neuro-
nal circuitry has demonstrated that synapses on somas and
dendrites can be modified according to their number (Fifkova
1970b; Globus et al 1973; Purpura 1974; Diamond et al 1975;
Cravioto et al 1976; Dyson & Jones 1976; Matthews et al
1976; Cotman & Lynch 1976; Pettegrew 1978; Roper & Ko 1978;
Pysh et al 1979), shape (Greenough et al 1978), size
(Fifkova 1970a, b; West & Greenough 1972; Diamond et al 1975;
Dyson & Jones 1976; Matthews et al 1976) and location
(Sotelo et al 1975; Berry & Bradley 1976; Sotelo &
Arsenio & Nunes 1976) as well as their source (Raisman 1969;
Llinas et al 1973; Changeux & Donchin 1977; Mariani et al
1977; Gall & Lynch 1978; Sotelo & Privat 1978). This
plasticity raises major questions as to possible mechanisms
responsible for organization of circuitry during development
and continual adjustment throughout life. The objective was
to determine if there were constant parameters which could
be related to factors that control organization of
circuitry (Hillman 1979).

In our studies on the reduction of numbers of afferent
synapses on Purkinje cells, synaptic size was quantitated
and compared to the number of afferents. An inverse relationship between the number of synapses and average size of
postsynaptic contact specializations resulted from a constant
total synaptic contact area on each Purkinje cell (Hillman
& Chen 1981b). This invariance in total synaptic area may
serve to stabilize synaptic input by allowing major shifts
in circuitry for developmental organization, learning and
compensation due to lesions and neuronal attrition.

METHODS

Afferents to Purkinje cells were reduced by either transection of parallel fibers in adult rats or reduction of
granule cells during development (induced by virus in newborn ferrets or malnutrition in the newborn rat). All animals were studied during adulthood for ultrastructural changes
in synaptic relationships in the molecular layer of the cerebellum. Quantitation of parallel fiber-Purkinje cell synaptic number and their contact length was achieved in the
malnutrition model by computer graphics methods.

Parallel Fiber Sectioning in the Adult Cerebellum

Parallel fibers were reduced in the rat by shallow single
or double transections across the longitudinal aspect of
folia. Single lesions were used to produce a gradient of
fiber reduction that was 50% or less. Greater than 50% reductions were induced by double lesions placed in line with
the parallel fiber bundles. These double cuts were spaced
at a 0.5 mm increment in the range of 0.5 to 2 mm. Single
lesions were made with a #11 surgical blade and double lesions
were made by separating two of the blades at specific distances with paraffin. All surgery was performed under a
dissecting binocular scope in order to ensure that the cuts
avoided large blood vessels and were maintained at less than
0.5 mm in depth.

In other groups of animals, a single folium was undercut
near its tip. A flattened 23 gauge needle was inserted very
obliquely along the longitudinal axis of a vermal folium extending from near the junction with the hemisphere of one
side toward the hemisphere on the other side. The zone of
the molecular layer, which overlay the granular layer
penetrated by the needle, was removed for study after perfusion for ultrastructure. This lesion resulted in transection
of parallel fibers and destruction of some granule cells,
thus, giving rise to reduction of parallel fibers within the
parallel fiber beam. This greatly reduced the number of
parallel fibers without destroying Purkinje cells in the zone
to be studied.

Animals were allowed to survive for varying periods of
time extending from one day to two months after which they
were anesthetized and perfused with phosphate buffered paraformaldehyde and glutaraldehyde.

Sagittal, 3 to 4 mm long, slices that were 0.5 mm thick
were removed from the area containing the lesion. Following
postfixation in osmium tetroxide and potassium ferrocyanide,
the tissue was block stained in uranyl acetate and then dehydrated and embedded in D.E.R. 332-732 epon. Semi-thin
sections that had hematomas or obvious Purkinje cell loss
were omitted. Control preparations were removed from the
contralateral folium at the same locations. Ultrathin
sections (50-60 nm) were analyzed on a JEOL 100C Electron
Microscope.

Agranular Ferret Cerebellum

Inoculation of newborn ferrets with panleucopenia
virus was used to reduce granule cell numbers for study of
afferent reductions to Purkinje cells (Llinas et al 1973).
Adult animals were sacrificed and prepared for ultrastructural observation as described above. Regions of the
vermis and hemispheres were sampled separately in order to
define the differences in synaptic size due to the reductions
in the number of parallel fibers in the molecular layer.

Malnutrition Induced Reduction of Granule Cells

Dietary protein restriction (8% for experimentals and
25% for control) with equal calories for both groups was
administered continuously from pregestation through lacta-
tion and to offspring until sacrifice at 60 days (Sterns
et al 1974). Light microscopic quantitation for volume
of the molecular layer, area of the Purkinje cell layer and
cell density were obtained from serially-sectioned brains.
Interactive and semi-automated, computer graphic techniques
were used to measure section area for volume of the molecular
layer, granule cell density, Purkinje cell density and area
of the Purkinje cell layer (Hillman et al 1977; Hillman &
Chen 1981a, b).

Ultrastructural sampling was done on the anterior
vermal folia and used to quantitate synaptic density and
size of synaptic contacts. Thin sections were sampled
throughout the width of the molecular layer by arbitrary
movement of the stage between the pia and the Purkinje cell
layer. The density of synapses in the molecular layer
was determined from the number of profiles and defined

stereologically by the method of Anker and Cragg (1974).
Total number of synapses in the molecular layer were obtained
from synaptic density and the volume of the molecular layer.
Four groups of animals were analyzed and considered separately
as male or female, control and experimental groups.

RESULTS

Qualitative Observations

    Ultrastructural observations on all 3 models of reduced
parallel fibers (two during development and one using parallel fiber sectioning in adult rats) revealed large spines
with elongated synaptic profiles (Figs. 1 & 2). Normal size
spines and giant spines were present in the same field.
Accompanying each enlarged spine was a much larger than normal parallel fiber bouton that had a proportional increase
in the number of synaptic vesicles in relation to their size.
Occasionally, two parallel fibers contacted the same spine.

    Postsynaptic thickenings were always opposed to presynap-
tic specialization sites. Many of the synaptic complexes
were found to circumscribe a major portion of the enlarged
spine (Figs. 1 & 2A) by a capping of the bouton. The length
of some of the synaptic profiles was obviously longer in
some preparations.

Parallel Fiber Reduction by Lesioning

    In single transections of folia, large synapses appeared
frequently near the lesion but were not visually discernable
at remote sites. With dual lesions of the folia, the size
of the spines and synapses were obviously increased as the
distances between the lesions was reduced. (Excessive trauma
also reduced the number of Purkinje cells; these preparations
lacked obvious changes in the size of spines and synapses).
A single transection with undercutting and involving the underlying granular layer produced giant spines by $2\frac{1}{2}$ days (Fig. 1).

    Besides the enlargement of spines, characteristic boutons
frequently encapsulated the enlarged spine heads. These
axonic enlargements contained at least the same proportion
of synaptic vesicles per unit area as the normal profiles.
Each enlarged spine had noticeable folds of endoplasmic

reticulum (ER) that were continuous with a single ER channel extending through the neck of the spine into the dendrites (Fig. 2A). Not all spines were enlarged, forming a mixed field of spine profile sizes (Fig. 2). In time sequence studies, the shift to larger spines was noted within 48 hours of the insult, and remained beyond the 2 month post-operative period that was studied.

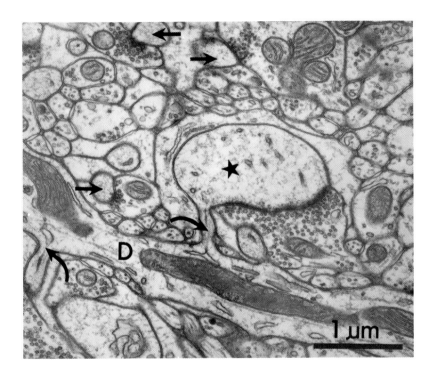

Fig. 1. Spine emerging from Purkinje cell dendrite makes an elongated synaptic contact with a parallel fiber bouton. Compare the normal sized spine (straight arrows) to the head of the giant spine (star) which is enlarged over 5 times in diameter. The spines are characterized by smooth endoplasmic reticulum which is continuous through the spine neck (curved arrows) with the endoplasmic reticulum in the dendritic shaft. A glial investment completely surrounds the spine and a portion of a parallel fiber bouton.

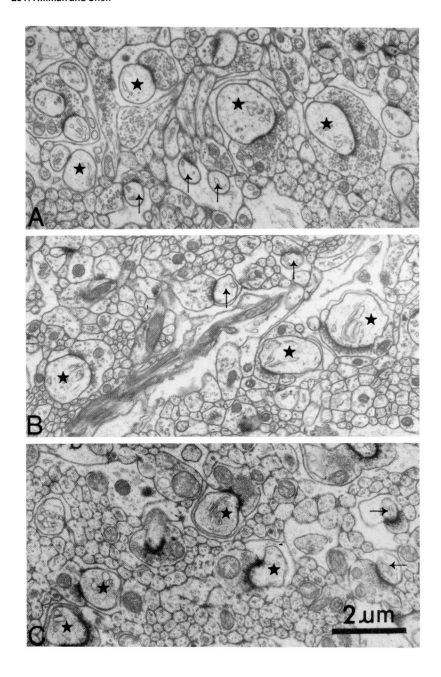

Virus-induced Parallel Fiber Reduction

Live virus inoculation of newborn animals that develop granule cells postnatally produced reductions in granule cell numbers (Margolis & Kilham 1968). Reinvestigation of the agranular cerebella (Llinas et al 1973) revealed enlarged spines in the cerebellar hemispheres in regions where granule cell numbers were not completely absent. Like parallel fiber sectioning, giant spines were common among normal-appearing spine processes that were making synaptic contacts. In those regions where parallel fibers were nearly absent, only occasional giant spines were seen among numerous spines having membrane thickenings but without presynaptic structures. These spine heads were encapsulated in glia. Like the other two models of afferent reduction, the parallel fiber boutons were enlarged and contained proportionally increased numbers of vesicles. Profiles of synaptic specializations were elongated and encapsulated much of the spine head.

Diet-Induced Parallel Fiber Reduction

Giant spines and elongated synaptic contacts were observed in the most severely affected female rat cerebella (Chen & Hillman 1980). Such spines had essentially the same characteristics as those produced in lesion and virus experiments.

The number of parallel fiber-Purkinje cell synapses was obtained by determination of molecular layer volume and synaptic density for Purkinje cell spines (Hillman & Chen 1981a, b). This analysis revealed five groups of animals - three female (with giant spines, without giant spines and controls) and two male groups (control and experimental). The total number of

Fig. 2. Giant spines (stars) from 3 models with decreased parallel fibers. Compare normal size spines (arrows) with the enlarged spine structures (stars). A) Molecular layer containing giant spines from undercut rat cerebellar folium. B) Molecular layer from malnourished female rat. C) Ferret cerebellum in regions of reduced granule cells. Note that the giant spines are similarly enlarged in all preparations. These spines have accompanying elongated synaptic clefts with a crown of synaptic vesicles. A massive core of endoplasmic reticulum is found in giant spines.

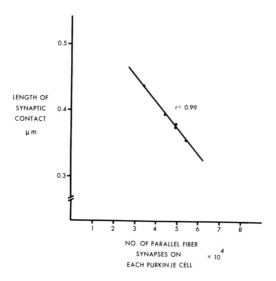

Fig. 3. Synaptic profile length and parallel
fiber synapses on Purkinje cells from five
groups of animals with degrees of granule cell
reduction. Line represents linear least-squares
fit determination and has a correlation coef-
ficient of 0.99

Table 1. Average Synaptic Profile Length,
Number of Spine Synapses and Their Total Area
of Contact on Each Purkinje Cell

	Number of Parallel Fiber Synapses on Each Purkinje Cell $(\times 10^4)$	Synaptic Profile Length (μm)	Total Synaptic Area on Each Purkinje Cell $(\mu m^2 \times 10^3)$
Female Control	5.40 (6)	0.355 ± 0.01 (7)	5.35
Female Deficient w/giant spines	3.42 (3)	0.436 ± 0.056 (3)	5.10
Female Deficient w/o Giant Spines	4.39 (8)	0.395 ± 0.014 (6)	5.36
Male Control	4.89 (6)	0.372 ± 0.016 (7)	5.33
Male Deficient	4.92 (5)	0.381 ± 0.022 (7)	5.61

( ) indicates the number of animals sampled

Purkinje cells remained the same in all groups. Determination of synaptic density and volume of the molecular layer
revealed that the number of synapses on each Purkinje cell
(the small percentage of climbing fibers was disregarded) was
reduced significantly in the deficient female group while
the males were virtually unchanged as compared to their controls. Since control males had fewer number of synapses
than control females, all four groups and a female subgroup
with obvious giant spines, had different numbers of synapses
on Purkinje cells (Table 1).

Length measurement for profiles of synaptic contacts revealed that average synaptic length was inversely related to
the number of parallel fiber synapses on each Purkinje cell
(Fig. 3; Table 1). For example, control females had the
largest number of synapses and the shortest average synaptic
profile length, while female animals with giant spines had
the smallest number of synapses but the greatest contact
length. Control males had a midrange-number of parallel fibers and had a midrange-average synaptic length (Table 1).
Determination of total contact area on each Purkinje cell
for these five groups revealed that the total synaptic contact area on each Purkinje cell did not vary more than $\pm$ 5%
(Table 1).

The shape and size of synapses between experimentals and
controls were further examined by 3-dimensional reconstruction. The shape of synaptic contacts was round to slightly
oval and formed a small flattened dome. Determination of
average area from this 3-dimensional data confirmed that
length determinations between synapses of different sizes
were adequate for estimating area since the overall curvatures
were, on the average, the same.

Discussion

Circuitry is constantly being modified during development, apparently by experience (Coss & Globus 1978; Floeter
& Greenough 1979; Pysh & Weiss 1979) as well as by other extrinsic influences (West & Kemper 1976; Pysh et al 1979;
Hillman & Chen 1981a) and aging (Buell & Coleman 1979). These
changes occur in varying degrees and, in some cases, without
notable consequence. Plasticity of circuitry has been documented to occur naturally (genetic mutations) or following
an array of induction methods ranging from traumatic lesions

(Cotman & Nadler 1978) to chemical inflictions (Sotelo et al 1975). The purpose of plasticity has been seen by many investigators as a method for maintenance of synaptic number. In other studies, synaptic size (Fifkova 1970a; Diamond et al 1975; Matthew et al 1976) and shape (Greenough et al 1978) changes have also been noted, but have received much less attention as elements of plasticity.

Circuitry Modification Following Reduced Afferents

Reduction in the number of afferents to an array of neuronal types has been produced by varied approaches both during development and in the adult. Early studies on the spinal cord (Lui & Chambers 1958) and data on the septal region (Raisman 1969) produced the basis of reactive synaptogenesis, suggesting that other afferent processes in the region take over synaptic sites. More recently, others have shown plasticity, such as the olfactory system (Graziadei & Graziadei 1978), red nucleus (Tsukahara 1978), sympathetic ganglion (Roper & Ko 1978) and hippocampus (Cotman & Nadler 1978).

Beside traumatic lesions, environmental conditions were also found to alter circuitry. In the visual system, dark vs. light rearing as well as altered visual patterns resulted in detectable modifications to afferent organization (Hubel & Weisel 1970; see also Pettegrew 1978). In comparisons between enriched and impoverished environments, measurements of synaptic contact length revealed smaller synaptic contacts in impoverished groups (West & Greenough 1972). A number of other indicators of synaptic relationships have been analyzed on Golgi preparations such as spine size, length and number (Purpura 1974; Coss & Globus 1978; Pysh et al 1979).

Elongation and enlargement of spines have been observed in agranular cerebella following x-irradiation at birth (Berry & Bradley 1976) as well as in genetic mutants (Sotelo 1975; Mariani et al 1977). The majority of Purkinje cell spines in agranular cerebella were near normal size and had postsynaptic densities which lacked presynaptic contact (Llinas et al 1973; Sotelo 1975a). On the contrary, in the cerebellum of Staggerer mutants, unusually long memebrane specializations resembling postsynaptic sites were found on dendritic shafts (Sotelo 1973). The Staggerer cerebellum may represent a defect in distribution in synaptic membrane molecules from the soma to synaptic insertion sites.

Following parallel fiber transsections, increased numbers of vesicles were apparent in enlarged parallel fiber
boutons. However, changes in spine size and synapses were
not noted by Mouren-Mathieu & Colonnier (1969). Elongated
synaptic junctions may not have been noticed because a small
change in contact diameter is actually a large change in contact area because of the exponential relationship. Furthermore, multiple sections through each synapse give rise to a
number of different profile sizes and thus reduce the possibility for qualitative comparisons.

Malnutrition produced alterations in Purkinje cell dendritic structures (West & Kemper 1976; McConnell & Berry 1979;
Pysh et al 1979) which were presumably due to the reduction
of afferents to these cells. Synaptic spines were markedly
enlarged in some of the most severely affected female animals
(Chen & Hillman 1980). The length of synaptic contacts on
these large spines was greatly elongated. Measurement of
synaptic size was necessary in order to determine differences
in contact area when afferent number was reduced (Hillman &
Chen 1981b).

Number of Synapses vs. Size of Synapses

Quantitation of synaptic density and length of synapses
in general revealed an inverse relationship between their
length and number. West and Greenough (1972) first demonstrated that the length of synaptic contacts was as much as
20% shorter under impoverished conditions as compared to complex environments. Later Diamond et al (1975) demonstrated
that the length change was between control and impoverished
groups and, furthermore, determined that synaptic density
increased as synaptic length decreased. This 11% increase
in density was accompanied by 6% reduction in length in
the impoverished group. Fifkova (1970a), studying deprivation
of light from birth, defined a 21% decrease in synaptic density which was accompanied by a 9% increase in synaptic
lengths in the visual cortex. Even greater reductions in
synaptic number were found in the lateral geniculate and were
accompanied by even greater increases in synaptic length
(Cragg 1969). Following undercutting of the cortex, Rutledge
(1978) reported as much as 20% reduction in synapses and a
5% increase in synaptic length. Lesions in the hippocampal
pathways produced a 13% increase in synaptic length and a
20% reduction in numbers of synapses in the outer two thirds

of the dentate gyrus following 205 days of recuperation
(Matthews et al 1976). All these studies lacked analysis of
volume for determination of the total number of synapses.
To our knowledge, the malnutrition study reported here is
the first to define the total number of synapses of a
particular type by both volume and density determinations.
We demonstrated that a similar inverse relationship occurred
with reduction of granule cell afferents to Purkinje cells
(Hillman & Chen 1981b). By the use of the ratio method,
differing degrees of afferent reductions had equally pro-
portioned increases in the average contact area of individual
synapses. Furthermore, these studies showed that the total
synaptic contact area remained constant for spine synapses
on each Purkinje cell regardless of the degree of afferent
reduction (Table 1).

The Purkinje cell circuitry represents a site where
there is limited competition for synaptic sites when parallel
fiber afferents are removed. Since parallel fibers make up
the majority of input to Purkinje cells, this leaves only
the single climbing fiber and remaining parallel fibers
(1:350) to compete for synaptic sites. The parallel fibers
evidently produce little competition since they do not
branch but remain in a single plane. These regenerating
afferents usually are blocked by the glia at the lesions
site. The single, branching climbing fiber can evidently
not assume a role in a massive takeover of synaptic sites.
Remaining parallel fibers that are immediately opposed to
Purkinje cell dendrites appear to develop new synaptic
contacts with spines (Chen & Hillman, unpublished results).
These new formations appear already at 2 days. With substantial loss of parallel fibers, the possibility of
parallel fibers contacting Purkinje cell dendrites is
reduced, resulting in profound increases in synaptic
contact size.

Constancy in Total Synaptic Contact Area for
Specific Receptor Types

At the molecular level, synaptic compensation can be
envisioned as a shift of synaptic location during the turnover period for postsynaptic membrane. If the production of
molecules is controlled by a system within the soma and then
transported to the receptor site (Altman 1971), a fairly
constant amount of postsynaptic macromolecules could regulate
a relatively constant total synaptic area. Since the smooth
ER may be the means of transportation for these molecules to

the dendritic sites, the distribution of ER could determine the position and even the size of certain synaptic types. Thus, a shift for receptor molecules would be to the remaining contact sites. In addition, there are some indications that synaptic size is limited and once this limit is reached, there is a tendency to develop perforations or multiple sites on the same dendritic area (Raisman & Field 1973; Matthew et al 1976; Cotman & Nadler 1978).

SUMMARY

Reduction of Purkinje cell afferents during development or after maturation resulted in a large change in the size of synaptic contacts on dendritic spines. Ultrastructural studies revealed enlarged Purkinje cell spines and elongation of the synapses with parallel fibers in three models of parallel fiber reduction: 1) developmental malnutrition, 2) developmental virus-induced granule cell reduction, and 3) parallel fiber sectioning in the adult. In developmental malnutrition, five groups of animals having different numbers of parallel fiber afferents to Purkinje cells, but the same total number of these cells, were quantitatively compared. As the number of synaptic junctions on Purkinje cells decreased, average area of synaptic contact increased. From this determination, it was further established that the total contact area on each Purkinje cell remained constant for groups of animals having different levels of afferent reduction. This inverse relationship was the result of Purkinje cells having a constant total synaptic contact area for parallel fibers. These studies show that the total postsynaptic area for each Purkinje cell is intrinsically determined and that synapses with the remaining parallel fibers change their size in a plastic response to interactions between pre- and postsynaptic elements.

REFERENCES

Altman J (1971). Coated vesicles and synaptogenesis. A developmental study in the cerebellar cortex of the rat. Brain Res. 311: 322.
Anker RL, Cragg BG (1974). Estimation of the number of synapses in a volume of nervous tissue from counts in thin sections by electron microscopy. J. Neurocytol. 3: 725-735.

Berry M, Bradley P (1976). The growth of the dendritic trees of Purkinje cells in irradiated agranular cerebellar cortex. Brain Res. 116: 361-387.

Bruell SJ, Coleman PD (1979). Dendritic growth in the aged human brain and failure of growth in senile dementia. Science 206: 854-856.

Changeux JP, Donchin A (1976). Selective stabilization of developing synapses as a mechanism for the specification of neuronal networks. Nature 264: 705-712.

Chen S, Hillman D (1980). Giant spines and enlarged synapses induced in Purkinje cells by malnutrition. Brain Res. 187: 487-493.

Coss R, Globus A (1978). Spine stems on tectal interneuron in Jewel fish are shortened by social stimulation. Science 200: 787-790.

Cotman CW, Lynch GS (1976). Reactive synaptogenesis in the adult nervous system: the effects of partial deafferentation on new synapse formation. In Barondes S (ed): "Neuronal Recognition", New York: Plenum Press, pp. 69-108.

Cotman CW, Nadler JV (1978). Reactive synaptogenesis in the hippocampus. In Cotman CW (ed): "Neuronal Plasticity", New York: Raven Press.

Cragg BG (1969). The effects of vision and dark-rearing on the size and density of synapses in the lateral geniculate measured by electron microscopy. Brain Res. 13: 53-67.

Cravioto HM, Randt CT, Derby BM, Diaz A (1976). A quantitative ultrastructural study of synapses in the brains of mice following early life undernutrition. Brain Res. 118: 304-306.

Diamond MC, Lindner B, Johnson R, Bennett EL, Rosenzweig MR (1975). Differences in occipital cortical synapses from environmentally enriched, impoverished and standard colony rats. J. Neurosci. Res. 1: 109-119.

Dyson SE, Jones DG (1976). Some effects of undernutrition on synaptic development. A quantitative ultrastructural study. Brain Res. 114: 365-378.

Fifkova E (1970a). The effect of molecular deprivation on the synaptic contacts of the visual cortex. J. Neurobiol. 1: 285-294.

Fifkova E (1970b). Changes of axosomatic synapses in the visual cortex of monocularly deprived rats. J. Neurobiol. 2: 61-72.

Floeter MK, Greenough WT (1979). Cerebellar plasticity: Modification of Purkinje cell structure by differential rearing in monkeys. Science 206: 227-229.

Gall C, Lynch G (1978). Rapid axon sprouting in the neonatal rat hippocampus. Brain Res. 153: 357-362.

Globus A, Rosenzweig MR, Bennett EL, Diamond MC (1973). Effects of differential experience on dendritic spine count. J. Comp. Physiol. Psych. 82: 175-181.

Gottlieb DI, Cowan WM (1972). Evidence for a temporal factor in the occupation of available synaptic sites during development of the dentate gyrus. Brain Res. 41: 452-456.

Graziadei PPC, Graziadei GAM (1978). The olfactory system: A model for the study of neurogenesis and axon regeneration in mammals. In Cotman CW (ed): "Neuronal Plasticity" New York: Raven Press.

Greenough WT, West RW, DeVoogd TJ (1978). Cerebellar plasticity: Modification of Purkinje cell structure by differential rearing in monkeys. Science 202:1096-1098.

Hillman DE (1979). Neuronal shape parameters and sub-structures as a basis of neuronal form. In Schmitt FO, Worden FG (eds): "The Neurosciences Fourth Study Program" Cambridge, Massachusetts and London: MIT Press, pp. 477-498.

Hillman DE, Chen S (1981a). Vulnerability of cerebellar development in malnutrition. I. Quantitation of layer volume and neuron numbers. In press.

Hillman DE, Chen S (1981b). Vulnerability of cerebellar development in malnutrition. II. Intrinsic determination of total synaptic area on Purkinje cell spines. In press.

Hillman DE, Llinás R, CHUJO M (1977). Automatic and semi-automatic analysis of nervous system structure. In Lindsay RD (ed): "Computer Analysis of Neuronal Structures", New York: Plenum Press, pp. 73-89.

Hubel DH, Wiesel TN (1970). The period of susceptibility to the physiological effects of unilateral eye closure in kittens. J. Physiol. 206: 419-436.

Liu CN, Chambers WW (1958). Intraspinal sprouting of the dorsal root axons. Arch. Neurol. (Chic.) 79: 46-61.

Llinás R, Hillman DE, Precht W (1973). Neuronal circuit reorganization in mammalian agranular cerebellar cortex. J. Neurobiol. 4: 69-94.

Margolis G, Kilham L (1968). In pursuit of an ataxic hamster, or virus-induced cerebellar hypoplasia. In "The Central Nervous System, International Academy of Pathology Monograph No. 9, U.S. Govt. Printing Office, Washington, D.C., pp. 157-183.

Mariani J, Crepel F, Mikoshiba K, Changeux JP, Sotelo C
    (1977). Anatomical, physiological and biochemical
    studies of the cerebellum from reeler mutant mouse.
    Phil Trans. B, 281: 1-28.
McConnell P, Berry M (1978) The effects of undernutrition
    on Purkinje cell dendritic growth in the rat.
    J. Comp. Neurol. 177: 159-172.
Matthews D, Cotman C, Lynch G (1976). An electron
    microscopic study of lesion induced synaptogenesis in
    the dentate gyrus of the adult rat. II. Reappearance
    of morphologically normal synaptic contacts.
    Brain Res. 115: 23-41.
Mouren-Mathieu AM, Colonnier M (1969). The molecular
    layer of the adult cat cerebellar cortex after lesion
    of the parallel fibers: An optic and electron microscope
    study. Brain Res. 16: 307-323.
Pettegrew JD (1978). The paradox of the critical period
    for striate cortex. In Cotman CW (Ed): "Neuronal
    Plasticity", New York: Raven Press, pp. 311-329.
Pysh JJ, Perkins RE, Beck LS (1979). The effect of post-
    natal undernutrition on the development of the mouse
    Purkinje cell dendritic tree. Brain Res. 163: 165-170.
Pysh JJ, Weiss GM (1979). Exercise during development
    induces an increase in Purkinje cell dendritic tree
    size. Science 206: 230-231.
Purpura DP (1974). Dendritic spine dysgenesis and mental
    retardation. Science 186: 1126-1128.
Raisman G (1969). Neuronal plasticity in the septal nuclei
    of the adult rat. Brain Res. 14: 25-48.
Raisman G, Field P (1973). A quantitative investigation
    of the development of collateral reinnervation after
    partial deafferentation of the septal nuclei.
    Brain Res. 50: 241-264.
Roper S, Ko C-P (1978). Synaptic remodeling in the
    partially denervated parasympathetic ganglion in the
    heart of the frog. In Cotman CW (ed): "Neuronal
    Plasticity", New York: Raven Press, pp. 1-25.
Rutledge LT (1978). Effects of cortical denervation and
    stimulation on axons, dendrites and synapses. In
    Cotman CW (ed): "Neuronal Plasticity", New York:
    Raven Press.
Sotelo C (1973) Permanence and fate of paramembranous
    synaptic specialization in mutant and experimental
    animals. Brain Res. 62: 345-351.
Sotelo C (1975a). Anatomical physiological and biochemical
    studies of the cerebellum from mutant mice. II.
    Morphological study of cerebellar cortical neurons and
    circuits in the Weaver mouse. Brain Res. 94: 9-44.

Sotelo C (1975b). Synaptic remodeling in mutants and experimental animals. In Vital-Durand F, Jeannerod M (eds): "Aspects of Neural Plasticity", Vol. 43, pp. 167-190.

Sotelo C, Arsenio-Nunes ML (1976). Development of Purkinje cells in absence of climbing fibers. Brain Res. 111: 389-395.

Sotelo C, Hillman DE, Zamora AJ, Llinas R (1975). Climbing fiber deafferentation: its action on Purkinje cell dendritic spines. Brain Res. 98: 574-581.

Sotelo C, Privat A (1978). Synaptic remodeling of the cerebellar circuitry in mutant mice and experimental cerebellar malformations. Acta Neuropathol. (Berl). 43: 19-34.

Stern W, Forbes WB, Resnick O, Morgane PJ (1974). Seizure susceptibility and brain amine levels following protein malnutrition during development in the rat. Brain Res. 89: 375-384.

Tsukahara N (1978). Synaptic plasticity in the red nucleus. In Cotman CW (ed): "Neuronal Plasticity", New York: Raven Press, pp. 113-130.

West RW, Greenough WT (1972). Effect of environmental complexity on cortical synapse of rats: Preliminary results. Behav. Biol. 7: 279-284.

West CD, Kemper TL (1976). The effect of a low protein diet on the anatomical development of the rat brain. Brain Res. 107: 221-237.

MORPHOLOGICAL BASIS OF
NEUROPHYSIOLOGY OF THE CEREBELLUM

Eleventh International Congress of Anatomy:
Glial and Neuronal Cell Biology, pages 249—258
© 1981 Alan R. Liss, Inc., 150 Fifth Avenue, New York, NY 10011

TRANSMISSION AND SCANNING ELECTRON MICROSCOPY AND ULTRACYTO-CHEMISTRY OF VERTEBRATE AND HUMAN CEREBELLAR CORTEX

Orlando J. Castejón and Haydée V. Castejón

Unidad de Investigaciones Biológicas. Facultad de Medicina. Universidad del Zulia. Apartado 526. Maracaibo. Venezuela.

The cerebellar cortex is an excellent and relatively simple model of the central nervous system which can be explored with the new techniques of electron microscopy and ultracytochemistry. In our laboratories, we have studied in the last sixteen years the cytoarchitectonic arrangement, neuronal circuits and acid polysaccharide histochemistry of the cerebellar cortex of different vertebrates including man in order to obtain further information and new knowledge on brain organization and to correlate morphological data and chemical composition of nervous transmission.

For transmission electron microscopy (TEM), cerebellum of adult normal albino mice, teleost fishes and men were used. The mouse and fish cerebellar cortex was fixed either by immersion or vascular perfusion with buffered glutaraldehyde phosphate solution and post-fixed with osmium tetroxide. The human cerebellum was obtained by surgical biopsy from patients with cerebellar tumors, brain trauma and vascular anomalies.

For the TEM ultracytochemical study (Castejón and Castejón, 1976) mouse cerebellar cortex was fixed by glutaraldehyde and then treated according to the following procedures:
a) Small blocks were post-fixed in osmium tetroxide followed by conventional TEM techniques.
b) Others were embedded in warm agar, sectioned 30 μm thick and then immersed in Alcian Blue (AB) staining solution, post-fixed in osmium tetroxide and embedded in araldite;

ultrathin sections were stained by uranyl and lead salts (GABOUL method).

c) Some parallel 30 μm sections of (b), previous to AB staining were incubated in either testicular hyaluronidase, neuraminidase or ribonuclease with their respective controls.

d) Some blocks of glutaraldehyde fixed tissue, without any further treatment, were dehydrated and embedded in araldite. Ultrathin sections were stained with the osmium coordination compound Os-DMEDA (Castejón and Castejón, 1972b).

For the scanning electron microscope (SEM), samples of fish and human cerebellar cortex, the latter obtained from autopsy material, were fixed 2-16 hours in 4% buffered glutaraldehyde, dehydrated through ethanol, frozen in liquid nitrogen and cryofractured with a pre-cooled razor blade (Humphreys et al., 1975). The critical point drying was done with liquid CO_2 followed by coating with a thin layer of gold-palladium.

Granule Cell Layer

The spheric or ovoid granule cells appeared in groups of four to eight. They exhibited a smooth surface in teleost fishes and a rough surface in humans, due to retraction induced by anoxic or post-mortem changes. Granule cell dendrites showed their typical claw-like endings establishing asymmetric or Gray's type I synaptic contacts with the mossy fiber rosettes (Fig. 1). The dendritic digits displayed a serrated edge making the "gearing type" synaptic connections as described by Cajal (1955). The filiform granule cell axons emerge directly from the cell body and ascend to the molecular layer making cruciform "en passant" Gray's type I synaptic contacts with Purkinje dendritic spines (Figs. 9, 12).

The ultracytochemical study revealed at the presynaptic axoplasm of mossy fiber rosettes a GABOUL and Os-DMEDA positive electron dense material surrounding synaptic vesicles and continuous with presynaptic dense projections (Figs. 2,3). This material was resistant to neuraminidase and ribonuclease and sensible to hyaluronidase (Fig. 4). These findings permit us to conclude that the axoplasmic material of mossy fiber endings is constituted by proteoglycans in which hyaluronic acid and/or chondroitin 4-and/or 6-sulphate are present (Castejón and Castejón, 1976).

At the SEM level, the Golgi cells (Fig. 5) are distinguished among groups of granule cells by their large size, horizontal and ascending dendrites and typical axonic arborization. The cryofracture method permitted the isolation of this neuronal type facilitating the integral visualization of the neuronal body and its processes. The Golgi cell axonic plexuses showed their characteristic constrictions and dilations and could be observed surrounding the glomerular islands.

The climbing fibers and their Scheibel's collaterals were also characterized in the granular and molecular layers of fish and human cerebellum (Fig. 7). They have a meandering course or spiral appearance and showed small collateral

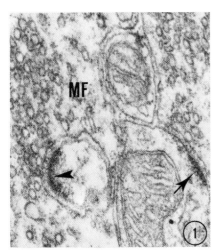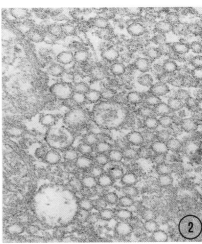

Fig. 1. Transmission electron micrograph of mouse mossy fiber-granule cell synaptic relationship. The mossy fiber (MF) rosette contains numerous clear, spheroidal synaptic vesicles. The arrowheads point out the asymmetric synaptic contact. The arrow indicates the synapse between a Golgi axonal ending and a granule cell dendrite. X 72 000.

Fig. 2. Transmission electron micrograph of mouse cerebellar cortex fixed by vascular perfusion with Alcian Blue-glutaraldehyde buffer phosphate solution. An alcianophilic material appears in the matrix of mossy fiber rosette, surrounding the clear, spheroidal synaptic vesicles. X 120 000.

excrescences and terminal boutons. These features allow a clear differentiation from the mossy fibers, which on the contrary displayed the rosette expansions.

In teleost cerebellar cortex, a clear distinction could be made at the SEM level between mossy and climbing fiber glomeruli (Castejón and Caraballo, 1980). The mossy fiber branches appeared as thick processes which send out small collaterals ending in a large granule. The mossy glomerular regions (Fig. 6) appeared as balls of yarn or entangled threads, polygonal, round or ovoid in shape, formed by the convergence of many dendritic processes (up to 18) of granule and Golgi cells upon the mossy fiber rosette. The mossy fiber emerges from the glomerulus and can be traced for a short distance to penetrate again into a neighbouring glomerulus. This observation confirms the "en passant" type of mossy fiber synaptic contacts. The climbing fiber glomeruli,

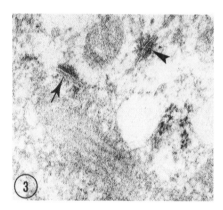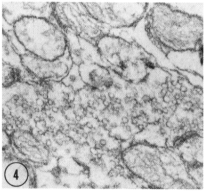

Fig. 3. Transmission electron micrograph of mouse cerebellar cortex. Os-DMEDA staining. An electron dense material is observed in the matrix of mossy fiber ending. The arrow points out the increased electron density of postsynaptic thickening. Similar features are observed at the dendrodendritic junction (arrowhead). X 60000.

Fig. 4. Transmission electron micrograph of mouse cerebellar cortex. Testicular hyaluronidase treatment of glutaraldehyde fixed mossy fiber ending followed by Alcian Blue staining. Note the disappearance of axoplasmic material after enzymatic treatment. X 60000.

first described by Palay and Chan-Palay (1974), appeared as thin, elongated or triangular structures (Fig. 7), where the climbing glomerular collateral appears surrounded by the granule cell dendritic digits (Fig. 7).In addition, climbing fiber showed fine tendril collaterals, characterized by varicosities or globular enlargements connected by a fine thread. Golgi cell axonal plexuses were observed participating in the formation of both glomerular types. Remnants of a neuroglial envelope were found in the mossy glomeruli but not in the climbing fiber glomeruli.

Purkinje Cell Layer

With TEM, teleost Purkinje cells (Fig. 8) showed a high ly electron dense material in the smooth endoplasmic

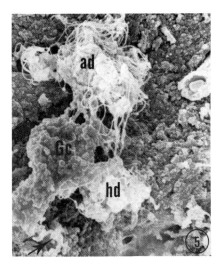 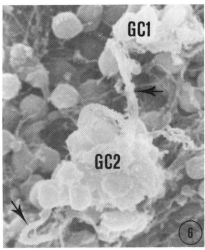

Fig. 5. Scanning electron fractograph of human cerebellar cortex. The cryofracture process isolated the Golgi cell allowing us to visualize the Golgi cell body (Gc), and its horizontal (hd), hairy ascending dendrites (ad) axonal plex us (arrow). A capillary is also seen. X 2 250.

Fig. 6. Scanning electron micrograph of fish mossy glomerular region. A mossy fiber (arrows) appears entering in two succesive granule cell groups (GC1,GC2) making "en passant" contacts. X 1 125.

reticulum, which appeared as membrane bound dense rods ran
domly distributed in the cytoplasm, dendritic arborization
and dendritic spines. The electron microscope images give
the impression that this osmiophilic substance arises from
the Golgi complex and later migrates toward the dendritic
processes to be incorporated into the post-synaptic density,
which is also considerably thickened. These dense rods have
not been yet observed in the Purkinje cells of other vertebrates (Caraballo and Castejón, 1979).

With the GABOUL method, the triple-layered structure
of Purkinje cell membrane was notably stained; a high electron dense inner and outer fuzzy coat was seen, increasing
the overall thickness of this membrane and making the Purkinje dendritic profiles more relevant than those of parallel fibers and Bergmann glial cell processes (Fig. 9). The

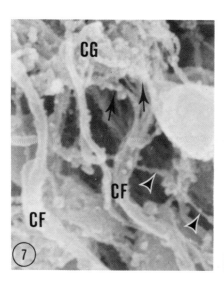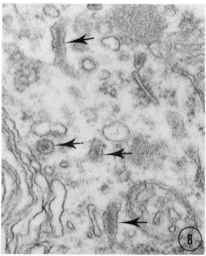

Fig. 7. Sagittal scanning electron micrograph of a fish
climbing fiber glomerulus (CG).Thick climbing fibers (CF)and
their thin collateral processes appear making synapses with
granule cell dendrites (arrows).The tendril collaterals of
climbing fibers are also visualized (arrowheads). X 3 500.
Fig. 8.Transmission electron micrograph of teleost Purkinje
cell cytoplasm showing dense rods (arrows) in the Golgi
region. X 60 000.

inner coating exhibited also short projections toward the
cytoplasmic matrix. No stainable material was seen in the
extracellular space between Purkinje cell membrane and Berg
mann glial cell membrane, the latter showed poor or no stain
ing. These findings reveal a different polysaccharide composition of both membranes (Castejón and Castejón, 1972a).

With GABOUL and Os-DMEDA the cytoplasmic matrix of
Golgi and Purkinje cells was densely stained,preferentially
between the cisternae of rough endoplasmic reticulum. A
close examination of this area showed irregular masses of

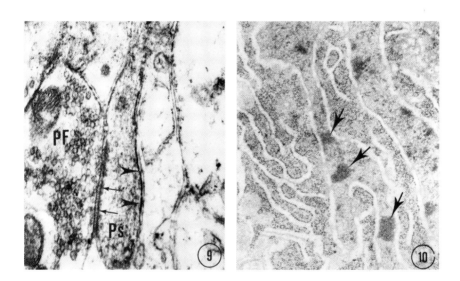

Fig. 9. Mouse cerebellar cortex fixed by vascular perfusion
with glutaraldehyde-Alcian Blue solution. Observe the dark
staining of Purkinje dendritic membrane (arrowheads) whereas
the apposed Bergmann glial cell membrane appears almost unstained. A parallel fiber (PF) is making asymmetric synaptic
contact with Purkinje dendritic spine (Ps). The postsynaptic
thickening (arrows) show a high electron density. X 60 000.
Fig. 10. Mouse cerebellar cortex fixed by glutaraldehyde
and stained on gold grids by the coordination compound
Os-DMEDA. The Golgi cell cytoplasm shows dark patches(arrows)
between the rough endoplasmic reticulum cisternae. X 30 000.

a high electron density dispersed throughout the cytoplasm
(Fig. 10). On the contrary, the neighbouring Bergmann glial
cell was not stained by the Os-DMEDA reagent. This finding
suggests the presence of chondroitin sulphate in the hyaloplasmic matrix of these macroneurons (Castejón and Castejón,
1972b).

With the SEM, the Purkinje cell body (Fig. 11) appeared
triangular or round in shape and showed an irregular, rough
surface. The fracture surface was produced at the level of
the neuroglial sheath, which almost completely covers the
Purkinje cells. Dark spaces were observed in the sites previously occupied by the Bergmann glial cells. The selective
removal of neuroglial cells allowed us to visualize the su-
pra and infraganglionic plexuses formed by the terminal arborization of the descending collaterals of basket cell axons and recurrent collaterals of Purkinje cell axons (Caste
jón and Valero, 1980).

The Molecular Layer

The SEM and cryofracture techniques provide a true ap-
preciation of the three-dimensional configuration of the Pur
kinje dendritic branches. In some fracture surfaces the Purkinje primary dendritic trunk could be observed projecting
vertically and devoid of the neighbouring molecular layer.
The surface of the trunk showed attachment of small and fine
processes, presumably corresponding to remaining neuroglial
cytoplasm and synaptic endings of climbing fibers and basket
cell axons. Purkinje secondary and tertiary dendritic branch
lets were observed ascending or curling downwards in the molecular layer. The parallel fibers (Fig. 12) were frequently
observed as bundles of fine threads passing in a perpendicu-
lar direction through the dendritic trees of the successive
Purkinje, stellate, basket and Golgi cells.

The stellate neurons exhibited short dendrites spreading into the molecular layer and filiform axons directed to
ward the neighbouring Purkinje dendritic branchlets.

At the TEM level, the fusiform thickenings of the parallel fibers were observed establishing Gray's type I synapt
ic connections with the Purkinje cell dendritic spines (Fig.
9). The spine synapses are completely surrounded by Bergmann
astrocytic cytoplasm. The morphology of the Purkinje

dendritic spines varies according to the species studied.The mouse and human spines showed a large neck in comparison to teleost spines, which appeared as neckless structures.

Alcian Blue staining showed clear and dark presynaptic terminals in the molecular layer. The clear types were seen in the parallel fiber-Purkinje spine synapses and axosomat- ic synapses of stellate neurons. The dark ones were found in some axosomatic contacts on stellate neurons and in the axodendritic contacts of stellate cell axons with Purkinje

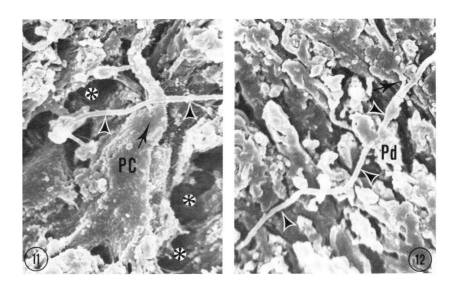

Fig. 11.Sagittal scanning electron fractograph of human cere bellar cortex. The Purkinje cell (PC) displays a pyriform shape and an anfractuous surface. The Bergmann glial cell and the Purkinje neuroglial sheath have been removed by the cryo fracture process. Dark spaces (asterisks) are observed at the sites previously occupied by these structures.The arrow indicate the emergence of the primary dendritic trunk. A bas ket cell axon is observed (arrowheads) running transversely across the upper pole of Purkinje cell soma. X 2 250.
Fig. 12.Transverse fractograph of human cerebellar cortex. A parallel fiber (arrowheads) is observed making "en passant" synaptic contact with sucessive Purkinje cell dendrites (Pd). The arrow points out an axospinodendritic contact. X 2 250.

dendrites. The dark presynaptic endings exhibited masses of
electron dense material dispersed throughout the axoplasmic
matrix and also a homogeneous dense substance surrounding
the synaptic vesicles. An increased electron density of the
synaptic complexes was also found. These latter findings reveal the synaptic localization of acid mucopolysaccharide-
Alcian Blue osmiophilic complexes (Castejón and Castejón,
1972a).

References

Cajal SR (1955). "Histologie de Systeme Nerveux de l'Homme
    et des Vertébrés". Vol II Madrid: Cons Sup Inv Cientif
    p 42.
Caraballo AJ, Castejón OJ (1979). Presence of dense rods in
    Purkinje cells of cerebellum of the Arius spixii. Morfol
    Normal Patol 3: 675.
Castejón HV, Castejón OJ (1972a). Application of Alcian
    Blue and Os-DMEDA in the electronhistochemical study of
    the cerebellar cortex I Alcian Blue staining. Rev Micros
    Elec 1: 207.
Castejón HV, Castejón OJ (1976). Electron microscopic demon
    stration of hyaluronidase sensible proteoglycans at the
    presynaptic area in mouse cerebellar cortex. Acta Histo-
    chem 55: 300.
Castejón OJ, Castejón HV (1972b). Application of Alcian
    Blue and Os-DMEDA in the electronhistochemical study of
    the cerebellar cortex II Os-DMEDA staining. Rev Micros
    Elec 1: 227.
Castejón OJ, Caraballo AJ (1980). Light and scanning elec-
    tron microscopic study of cerebellar cortex of teleost
    fishes. Cell Tissue Res 207: 211.
Castejón OJ, Valero CJ (1980). Scanning electron microscopy
    of human cerebellar cortex. Cell Tissue Res In Press.
Humphreys WJ, Spurlock BO, Johnson JS (1975). Transmission
    electron microscopy of tissue prepared for scanning elec-
    tron microscopy by ethanol-cryofracturing. Stain Tech 50:
    119.
Palay SL, Chan-Palay V (1974). "Cerebellar Cortex. Cytology
    and Organization". Berlin: Springer-Verlag p 287.

Eleventh International Congress of Anatomy:
Glial and Neuronal Cell Biology, pages 259—268
© **1981 Alan R. Liss, Inc., 150 Fifth Avenue, New York, NY 10011**

STRUCTURE AND FIBER CONNECTIONS OF THE CEREBELLUM

J. Voogd[x], F. Bigaré[x], N.M. Gerrits,
and E. Marani
Dpt. of Anatomy, University of Leiden, The
Netherlands and[x] Dpt. of Anatomy, Free University
of Brussels V.U.B., Belgium
Wassenaarseweg 62, 2333 AL Leiden, The Netherlands

The variations in gross morphology of the cerebellum contrast with the uniform histology of its cortex. In many investigations the borders between the cerebellar lobes and
lobules were considered as the natural boundaries for afferent and efferent fiber connections of the cerebellum. However,
many fiber systems do not terminate in, or originate from,
specific lobules, but are connected with longitudinal cortical zones, which often are continuous through several successive lobules. This longitudinal arrangement of the fiber connections of the cerebellum proved to be characteristic for
the efferent connections of the Purkinje cells with the central nuclei and for their climbing fiber afferents from the
contralateral inferior olive (fig. 1). For the mossy fiber
systems, which originate from multiple sources in the cord,
and the brain stem and which terminate in the granular layer,
a lobular organization prevails.

Purkinje cell fibers can be distinguished by their large
calibre (2-5 μm) from the mossy and the climbing fiber afferents which generally are smaller. In the cerebellar white
matter the fibers from Purkinje cells which project to certain central cerebellar nuclei collect in parallel sheets.
The sheets are separated by narrow spaces which are filled
with smaller, presumably afferent fibers. In Häggqvist stained sections the bundles of Purkinje cell fibers stain lighter
and the strips of small fibers show up as dark bands (the
"raphes", Voogd, 1964, fig. 3). A bundle of Purkinje cell
axons and the raphe which delimits it on its lateral side
are called a "compartment". The compartments in the cerebellar white matter can be reconstructed from serial sections

(fig. 2; Voogd and Bigaré, 1980).

    The hypothesis that the Purkinje cells, whose axons
use a certain compartment to terminate in a central cerebellar or vestibular nucleus, are located in discrete longitudinal zones in the cerebellar cortex, was tested in experiments in cats with injections of horseradish peroxidase
(HRP) in the central nuclei (Bigaré, 1980). The labeled
Purkinje cells were plotted in drawings of the sections,
and from these drawings graphical reconstructions of the
cerebellum were prepared, in which the superficially located Purkinje cells were indicated. Several of these experiments are illustrated in figure 4. After injections of
the posterior interposed nucleus a single band of labeled
Purkinje cells is present in the hemisphere of the anterior
lobe. This band (the C_2 zone) can be traced in the hemisphere
of the posterior lobe, into the ansiform lobule, the para-
median lobule, in the ventral part of the dorsal and in the
dorsal part of the ventral paraflocculus. The C_2 zone ends
in the medial part of the flocculus.

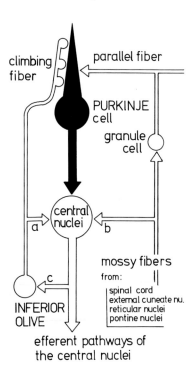

climbing fiber

parallel fiber

PURKINJE cell

granule cell

central nuclei

a   b

mossy fibers
from:
spinal cord
external cuneate nu.
reticular nuclei
pontine nuclei

c

INFERIOR OLIVE

efferent pathways of
the central nuclei

After injections of the anterior interposed nucleus two
bands of labeled cells (C_1
and C_3) are present on both
sides of the C_2 zone of the
previous experiment. In the
ventral part of the anterior
lobe the C_1 and C_3 zones fuse,
and in the posterior lobe they
do not reach beyond the para-
median lobule. Similar Purkinje
cell zones were seen after injections of the fastigial nucleus (the A zone), Deiters'
nucleus (the B zone) and the
caudal and rostral parts of the
lateral cerebellar nucleus (the
D_1 and D_2 zones). The localization of these zones is shown in

Fig. 1
Diagram showing the main fiber
connections of the cerebellum.

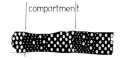

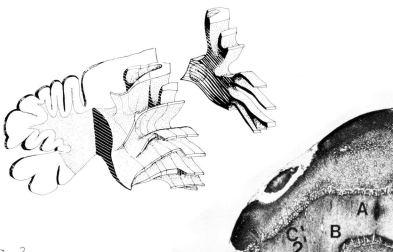

2

Fig. 2
Graphical reconstruction
of the white matter of
the anterior lobe of the
cerebellum of the ferret,
showing its division into
compartments. On the right
side a single compartment
with its central nucleus
is shown.

Fig. 3
Häggqvist stained sec-
tion through the anterior
lobe of the cat. Raphes
separate the compartments
A-C. (From Voogd and
Bigaré, 1980).

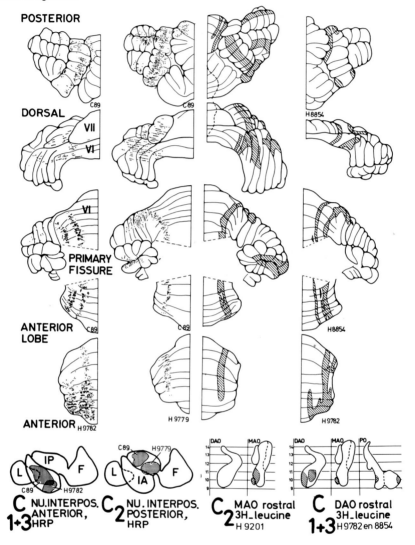

Fig. 4

Diagrams showing the localization of labeled Purkinje cells after injections of HRP in the anterior and posterior interposed nucleus, and identical localizations of the climbing fibers after injections of 3H-leucine in the accessory olives. From the top to the bottom diagrams depict caudal and dorsal views of the posterior lobe, the rostral and caudal banks of the primary fissure and a rostral view of the anterior lobe.

Fig. 5
Diagram showing the longitudinal
Purkinje cell zones projecting to
certain central cerebellar nuclei.
From top to bottom, a lateral view
of the cerebellum, and posterior
and dorsal views of the posterior
lobe are drawn, followed by the rostral and caudal banks of the primary
fissure and dorsal and rostral views
of the anterior lobe. At the bottom
the central nuclei are shown in the
same shadings as the zones (Bigaré,
1980).

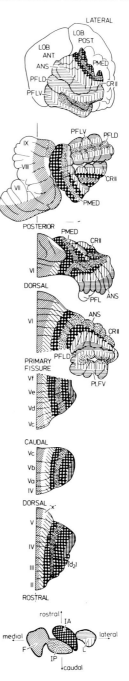

figure 5. In the vermis the A and B
zones are present, the hemisphere
consists of the C and D zones.

A similar longitudinal pattern
was found to be present in the termination of the olivocerebellar
climbing fiber system (Groenewegen
and Voogd, 1977; Groenewegen et al.,
1979). Fibers from certain parts of
the inferior olive traverse the compartments in the cerebellar white
matter in the reverse direction to
terminate with climbing fibers on
the longitudinal strips of Purkinje
cells. Olivocerebellar fibers moreover terminate with collaterals (a,
in fig. 1) on the central nucleus
located within the compartment.
Autoradiography of 3H-leucine injected into the inferior olive made
it possible to analyze this system
in detail. After injections into
the rostral half of the dorsal accessory olive (fig. 4) the C_1 and C_3
zones are labeled, after injections
in the rostral half of the medial
accessory olive labeling is found in
the C_2 zone and the posterior interposed nucleus (fig. 4 and 6).

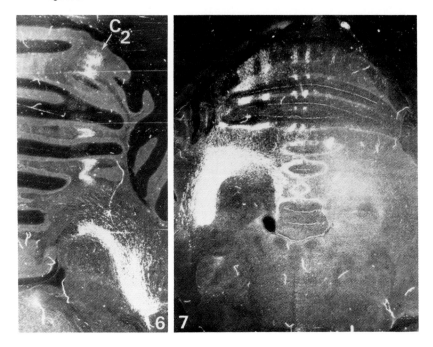

Fig. 6   Autoradiogram of the anterior lobe showing labeling
of the C_2 compartment and zone after an injection of
tritiated leucine in the medial accessory olive.

Fig. 7   Autoradiogram of the anterior lobe showing labeling
of patches of mossy fiber terminals in the granular
layer after an injection of tritiated leucine in the
external cuneate nucleus.

Climbing fibers to the A and B zones originate from caudal
halves of the medial and dorsal accessory olives respectively. The principal nucleus of the inferior olive gives rise
to the climbing fibers of the D zones (fig. 8).

The distribution of the terminals of mossy fiber systems
in the granular layer usually includes vermis and hemispheres
of certain cerebellar lobules. Collaterals of mossy fibers
moreover terminate in the central cerebellar nuclei (b, in
fig. 1). Within the projection area of a given mossy fiber
system a parcellation of the terminals is often visible in
parallel, longitudinal concentrations (fig. 7). In figure 9
the distribution of the terminals of certain mossy fiber

systems is illustrated in graphical reconstructions of the anterior surface of the anterior lobe and the rostral and caudal banks of the opened primary fissure (Gerrits, unpublished material; Gerrits and Voogd, 1979).

Spinocerebellar tracts were studied with degeneration techniques after partial lesions of the cord. The dorsal spinocerebellar tract, as depicted in figure 9, terminates bilaterally in the rostral and ventral part of the anterior lobe and in the bottom of the primary fissure. Fibers of the external cuneate nucleus were traced in autoradiograms after injections of tritiated amino acids in the external cuneate nucleus. This system terminates mainly ipsilaterally in the bottom of the primary fissure. Both systems show a marked longitudinal localization of their terminals. Reticulocerebellar fibers from the nucleus reticularis tegmenti pontis were also studied in autoradiographic material. They terminate in an overlapping manner with the former two mossy fiber systems, but terminate more heavily in the lateral part of the anterior lobe. In addition reticulocerebellar fibers terminate in circumscribed portions of all central nuclei. Collaterals of mossy fibers were not observed in the central nuclei in experiments on the spinocerebellar and cuneocerebellar tracts.

A longitudinal zonal distribution is present therefore in mossy fiber terminals in the granular layer, in climbing fiber terminals in the molecular layer and in the Purkinje cell axons in the cerebellar white matter. Marani and Voogd (1977) demonstrated an intrinsic longitudinal pattern in the distri-

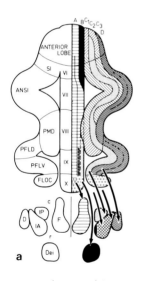

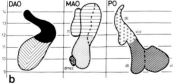

Fig. 8
Diagram of the olivocerebellar projection in the cat.
(Groenewegen et al., 1979).

NRTP **CE** **DSCT**

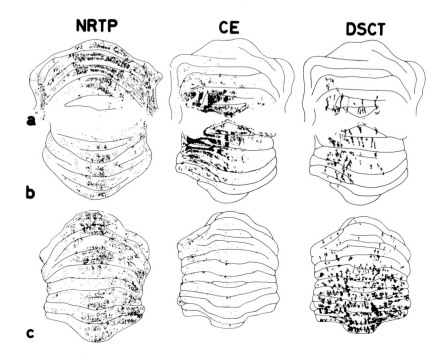

Fig. 9   The termination of certain mossy fiber systems in
the anterior lobe of the cat. From top to bottom the
diagrams indicate the caudal (a) and rostral (b)
banks of the opened primary fissure, and a rostral
view of the anterior lobe (c). Dots indicate mossy
fiber terminals plotted in the sections. From left to
right terminals from the nucleus reticularis tegmenti
pontis (NRTP), the external cuneate nucleus (CE) and
the dorsal spinocerebellar tract (DSCT) are shown.

bution of acetylcholinesterase (AChE) in the molecular layer.
In young cats till 4-5 months of age, bands of high AChE activity are present in the molecular layer of the vermis at
the midline, and in a position corresponding to the lateral
part of the A zone. The lateral part of the hemisphere is
uniformly positive for AChE. In older cats the entire molecu-

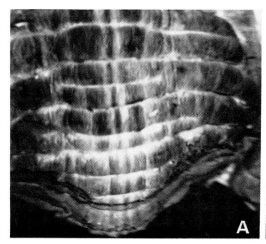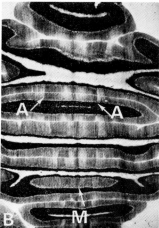

Fig. 10 A   Localization of the bands of high and low activity of AChE in the vermis of cat cerebellum. Whole mount preparation. Incubation according to Lewis and Knight (1977). Marani (unpublished).

Fig. 10 B   Localization of AChE in the molecular layer of cat cerebellum. Note accumulations at the midline and at the lateral border of the A zone. (Marani and Voogd, 1977b).

lar layer becomes negative for the enzyme. Ultrastructural histochemistry of AChE shows that the enzyme is present in parallel fibers and in Purkinje cell dendrites (Marani and Voogd, 1977a).

The longitudinal Purkinje cell zone with its corresponding nucleus and its connections with the inferior olive constitutes a functional unit. Through their efferent paths the units, or cerebellar modules, each exert an influence on a certain aspect of motor behaviour (Oscarsson, 1979). Association pathways between the modules appear to be absent. Integrated activity of the modules may be achieved through the mossy fiber-parallel fiber system, which has a mainly transverse orientation and always spans the width of several modules. In the parcellation of the mossy fiber terminals and in the periodicity in the distribution of AChE along the parallel fibers, this system also shows signs of a longitudinal organization.

REFERENCES

Bigaré F (1980). De efferente verbindingen van de cerebellaire schors van de kat. Thesis, Leiden University, The Netherlands.
Gerrits NM, Voogd J (1979). Cerebellar mossy fiber systems in the cat. Acta Morphol Neerl-Scand 17:236.
Groenewegen HJ, Voogd J (1977). The parasagittal zonation within the olivocerebellar projection. I Climbing fiber distribution in the vermis of cat cerebellum. J Comp Neur 174:417.
Groenewegen HJ, Voogd J, Freedman SL (1979). The parasagittal zonation within the olivocerebellar projection. II Climbing fiber distribution in the intermediate and hemispheric parts of cat cerebellum. J Comp Neur 183:551.
Lewis PR, Knight DP (1977). "Staining Methods for Sectioned Material". Amsterdam: North-Holland Publ Co.
Marani E, Voogd J (1977a). A longitudinal pattern of AChE in the molecular layer of the cerebellum of the cat. Acta Morph Neerl-Scand 15:332.
Marani E, Voogd J (1977b). An AChE band-pattern in the molecular layer of the cat cerebellum. J Anat 124:335.
Oscarsson O (1979). Functional units of the cerebellum - sagittal zones and microzones. TINS 2:143.
Voogd J (1964). The cerebellum of the cat. Thesis, Leiden University, The Netherlands. Assen: Van Gorcum and Co.
Voogd J, Bigaré F (1980). Topographical distribution of olivary and cortico nuclear fibers in the cerebellum: A review. In Courville J, De Montigny C, Lamarre Y (eds): "The Inferior Olivary Nucleus - Anatomy and Physiology", New York: Raven Press.

ABBREVIATIONS

ANS	ansiformis	IA	n. interpositus ant.
β	n. beta	IP	n. interpositus post.
CE	n. cuneatus ext.	L	n. cerebellaris lat.
CRII	Crus II	MAO	medial acc. olive
DAO	dorsal acc. olive	NRTP	n.retic.tegm. pontis
dc	dorsal cap	PFLD	paraflocculus dorsalis
Dei	n. Deiters	PFLV	paraflocculus ventralis
dl	dorsal leaf PO	PMED	(PMD) l. paramedianus
dmcc	dorsal medial cell col.	PO	principal olive
DSCT	dorsal spinocereb.tract	SI	l. simplex
F	n. fastigii	vl	ventral leaf PO
FLOC	flocculus	vlo	ventrolateral outgrowth

Eleventh International Congress of Anatomy:
Glial and Neuronal Cell Biology, pages 269–277
© 1981 Alan R. Liss, Inc., 150 Fifth Avenue, New York, NY 10011

MORPHOLOGICAL CORRELATES OF CEREBELLAR PURKINJE CELL
ACTIVITY

Jean C. DESCLIN, F.COLIN and J. MANIL

*Laboratories of Histology and of General Phy-
siology, ULB, Laboratorium voor Fysiologie en
Fysiopathologie, VUB, Brussels, Belgium.*

Establishing reliable morphological correlates of neuronal activity is one of our days' most formidable challen-
ges to students of CNS ultrastructure. Numerous studies
have provided, for example, a wealth of evidence strongly
suggesting that increased synaptic activity is reflected by
enhanced synaptic vesicle and plasma membrane recycling
(reviewed by Zimmerman, 1979). The microscopist's approach
to this problem in the mammalian CNS is fraught with many
difficulties such as, among others, the reliable ultrastructural identification of those very axon terminals belonging to neurons whose activity can be electrophysiolo-
gically assessed shortly before fixation.

Cerebellar Purkinje cells (PCs) should provide an especially favorable model for this kind of study. First,
they constitute a large and rather homogeneous neuronal population, cerebellar cortical and nuclear circuitries presently are among the best known, PC terminals form a majority among synapses on cerebellar nuclear neurons (Palay
and Chan-Palay, 1974; Chan-Palay, 1977). Second, electrical
activity of very large numbers or even of all PCs can be
predictably and dramatically altered for long periods of
time by simple experimental procedures.

Inferior olive (IO) destruction in rats recently was
shown to result almost immediately in a markedly enhanced
and very regular simple spike (SS) activity of PCs. Con-
versely, climbing fiber (CF) stimulation at frequencies
even as low as 2/sec resulted in almost complete suppression of the SS firing (Colin et al., 1980). Slow "on" and

"off" effects of CF activity on the SS firing were distinct
from and evolved on a much longer time scale than the classical 100-200 msec pauses following CF activity. It was
concluded from these data that CF stimulation reduces the
net activity of corresponding PCs and exerts on these cells
a powerful inhibitory influence. Hence, destruction of the
IO should provide a convenient means to durably increase
PC activity.

On the other hand, harmaline treatment was found to
selectively enhance IO activity, which resulted in a rhythmical activation of large numbers of cerebellar CFs
(De Montigny and Lamarre, 1973; Llinás and Volkind, 1973).
Effects of harmaline injections last more than 3 h in rats
and sustained CF rhythmical activity can be maintained for
long periods by injections repeated at intervals of 2 h.
Such experimental design should provide us with a situation fairly opposite to that resulting from IO destruction.

A recent ultrastructural study reported that numerous axon terminals of PCs abutting onto the nuclear neurons underwent a series of cytological changes in olivoprival rats (Desclin and Colin, 1980). About 2-3 h after the
death of IO neurons, PC boutons became filled with numerous
membrane-bounded vesicles and vacuoles. From 24 h onwards,
numerous PC endings became markedly depleted or even almost completely devoid of their synaptic vesicles. Even in
those boutons which apparently maintained their usual ultrastructure, numbers of synaptic vesicles seemed to be
lower than in controls. Objective assessment of this decrease required actual counts of synaptic vesicles in an adequate number of PC terminals from both experimental and
control animals.

PC axon endings in the cerebellar cortex and deep
nuclei were compared in electron micrographs from 3-acetyl-
pyridine (3-AP)-treated rats and from rats which had received 3 injections of harmaline (15 mg/kg, i.p.) at intervals of 2 h and were killed 1.5 h after the third injection. For our purpose, the latter experimental animals were
preferred to so-called "normal control rats". We assumed
that harmaline treatment should synchronize and homogenize
activities of most PCs, whereas the actual activities of
individual PCs from normal rats could only be guessed at.
Untreated rats were also used, however , in order to veri-
fy whether spontaneous alterations, if any, were not mis-

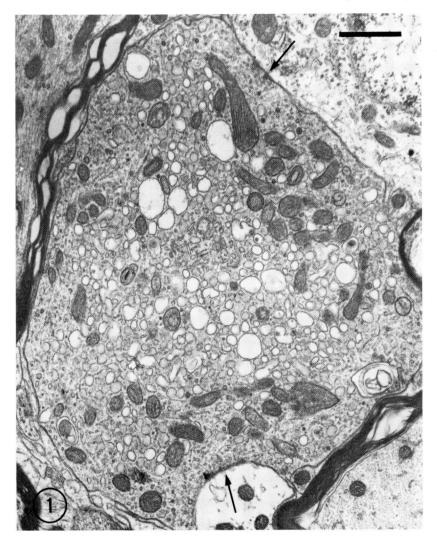

Fig. 1. This enlarged PC axon terminals makes synaptic
contact with a dendrite and a perikaryon (arrows). It
is filled with numerous membrane-bound vacuoles. 8 days
after 3-AP injection. Nucleus interpositus anterior.
Calibration : 1μm.

takenly attributed to treatments (Sotelo and Palay, 1971; Chan-Palay, 1973).

Electron micrographs of the cerebellar cortex and deep nuclei from 3-AP-treated rats were taken at survival times ranging from 2 h up to several months after the injection. PC axon terminals were identified according to ultrastructural features already described at length in the rat and other species (Larramendi and Lemkey-Johnston, 1970; Chan-Palay, 1971, 1977). First noticeable cytological changes undergone by these terminals became apparent from 9 h onwards after the treatment. These alterations were present in all central and Deiters' nuclei alike but required an additional 9 h to develop in the cortex. They consisted of the accumulation of membrane-bound vacuoles which seemed to be continuous with the smooth endoplasmic reticulum and appeared to distend the greatly enlarged terminals (Fig. 1). Such numerous and frequently huge vacuoles were present only in PC terminals, about 50 percent of these being affected in the nuclei during the first 3 days. Their frequency then gradually subsided, but they never completely disappeared, even at 6 months, whereas such pictures were exceedingly difficult to find in control animals.

From 24 h onwards, PC axonal boutons in the cortex (on Golgi and Lugaro cells) or contacting nuclear neurons became greatly enlarged (5-10µm diameter) and filled with an homogeneous finely granular material. Such terminals were markedly depleted or even devoid of synaptic vesicles. When present, the latter were as a rule clustered near the 'synaptic active zone' (Figs 3, 4) but sometimes a few persisting vesicles could also be found dispersed and suspended in the darkened axoplasm (Fig. 3). Although no statistical analysis has been performed, such greatly enlarged terminals, which could be identified even in plastic sections at light microscopic level, were frequently encountered in any grid from our experimental animals, whereas we found them only twice in 11 controls. Such depleted boutons were most frequent between 30 h and 8 days. Later on, they became less frequent but nervertheless were much more readily detected in olivoprival animals than in intact rats, even at 2 months.

Still another modification of PC axon terminals consecutive to IO destruction consisted of the accumulation of clustered small elliptical or flattened, membrane-bound

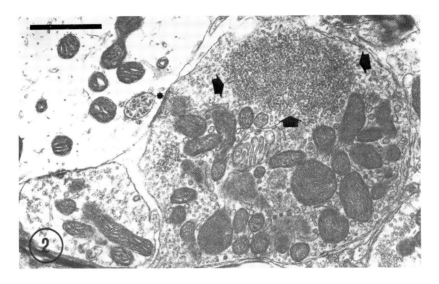

Fig. 2. Large clusters of small flattened vesicles closely packed together (large arrows) show up in PC terminals
consecutive to 3-AP treatment. N. interpositus anterior.
8 days survival. Calibration : 1 μm.

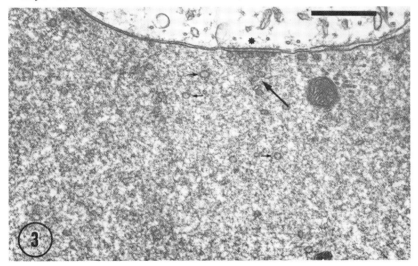

Fig. 3. Enlarged PC terminals are filled with a darkened
granular material with only few synaptic vesicles. N.
interpositus anterior. 8 days survival. Calibration :
0.5 μm.

vesicles showing up from 16 h onwards (Fig. 2). Their mean long axis was 43.33 + 0.35 nm in length (N = 615) whereas normal synaptic vesicles had a long axis measuring 59.28 + 0.48 nm (N = 328). About every third bouton of PC in any of the cerebellar nuclei contained such abnormal vesicles during the first week after 3-AP treatment. Then this frequency gradually decreased, but clusters of these organelles could still be consistently detected at 3 months.

Next, we counted vesicles in PC terminals in the nucleus interpositus anterior from 2 harmaline-treated rats (N = 85) and from 3 rats treated with 3-AP 24 h before the kill (N = 98). Hypertrophied terminals completely or markedly depleted of vesicles, or those containing swarms of small abnormal vesicles were excluded from these counts (in order to avoid ambiguities in identifying either terminals or synaptic vesicles). For harmaline-treated animals, 32093 vesicles were counted over a surface of 249.9 sq micra, which corresponded to a mean density of 128.4 vesicles/μm^2. In 3-AP-treated rats we found 17147 vesicles over 379.2 μm^2, i.e. a mean density of 45.2 vesicles/μm^2. Covariance analysis of these results (in order to reduce the variance due to varying sizes of measured profiles) showed these differences in densities of synaptic vesicles to be highly significant (F = 264.5, d.f. 1, 180). Thus, even when not taking into account those PC terminals which were obviously hypertrophied and almost devoid of synaptic vesicles, a clear decrease in numbers of synaptic vesicles emerged as a consequence of IO destruction.

In order to confer more general significance to these findings, comparisons between vesicle densities should also include untreated "control" rats. Work along these lines is presently in progress. However, preliminary results lead us to think that variability in vesicle density might be much higher in such rats, so that higher numbers of profiles should be measured and counted from more animals before obtaining significant figures.

It has been said above that IO destruction results in a markedly enhanced SS firing of PCs. Cytological changes described here are suggestive of an increased recycling of synaptic vesicles which would follow from such enhanced activity. Furthermore, the decrease in numbers of synaptic vesicles could also reflect a depletion of transmitter stores in PC terminals, which would be consis-

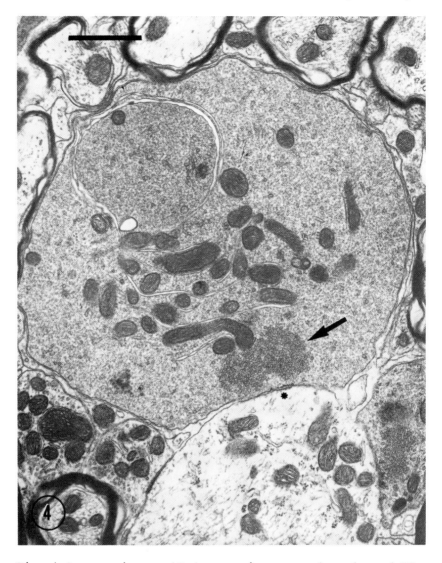

Fig. 4.Consecutive to IO destruction, greatly enlarged PC
terminals such as this one become quite frequent. Only few
synaptic vesicles cluster near the synaptic 'active' zone
(arrow). Mitochondria and cisterns of smooth reticulum are
present within the darkened and homogeneous axoplasmic
matrix. N. interpositus anterior. Survival: 8 days.
Calibration: 1 μm.

tent with the observation that synaptic efficiency of PCs is markedly reduced after IO destruction (Ito et al., 1978, 1979). This view is also supported by the evolution with time of the clinical picture of 3-AP-treated rats (Desclin and Colin, 1980): a first acute stage lasting for about 24 h reflected excessive PC activity resulting in inhibition of cerebellar and vestibular nuclei: animals were obviously hypotonic. During the following days, hypotonia gradually was replaced by hypertonia and ataxy. This was thought to reflect exhaustion of PC synaptic endings. In further support of this opinion came the observation that 3-AP treatment of colchicine-primed rats resulted in the immediate development of the decortication syndrome without any intermediate stage of hypotonia (Desclin and Colin, unpublished results).

Besides the decrease in numbers of synaptic vesicles, it remains at present undecided whether all observed ultrastructural changes should be ascribed to the enhanced PC firing alone. Some alterations already described by others (Sotelo and Palay, 1971; Chan-Palay, 1973) and mostly involving the smooth endoplasmic reticulum, were possibly slightly more frequent in our 3-AP-treated rats than in controls. As a working hypothesis, one might speculate that CF deafferentation also removes a trophic effect on the PCs (Ito et al., 1979), possibly by altering calcium currents at the level of PC dendrites (Llinás, 1979).

REFERENCES

Chan-Palay V (1971). The recurrent collaterals of Purkinje cell axons: A correlated study of the rat's cerebellar cortex with electron microscopy and the Golgi method. Z Anat Entwickl-Gesch 134:200.
Chan-Palay V (1973). Neuronal plasticity in the cerebellar cortex and lateral nucleus. Z Anat Entwickl-Gesch 142:23.
Chan-Palay V (1977). "Cerebellar Dentate Nucleus. Organization, Cytology and Transmitters." Berlin: Springer.
Colin F, Manil J, Desclin JC (1980). The olivocerebellar system I. Delayed and slow inhibitory effects: an overlooked salient feature of cerebellar climbing fibers. Brain Res 187:3.
De Montigny C, Lamarre Y (1973). Rhythmic activity induced by harmaline in the olivo-cerebello-bulbar system in the cat. Brain Res 53:81.

Desclin JC, Colin F (1980). The olivocerebellar system
II. Some ultrastructural correlates of inferior olive destruction in the rat. Brain Res 187:29.

Ito M, Orlov I, Shimoyama I (1978). Reduction of the cerebellar stimulus effect on rat Deiters neurons after chemical destruction of the inferior olive. Exp Rain Res
33:143.

Ito M, Nisimaru N, Shibuki K (1979). Destruction of inferior
olive induces rapid depression in synaptic action of cerebellar Purkinje cells. Nature (Lond) 227:568.

Larramendi LMH, Lemkey-Johnston NJ (1970). The distribution of recurrent Purkinje collateral synapses in the
mouse cerebellar cortex: an electron microscopic study.
J comp Neurol 138:451.

Llinás R (1979). The role of calcium in neuronal function.
In Schmitt FO, Worden FG (eds): "The Neurosciences:
Fourth Study Program", Cambridge MA: M.I.T. Press, p 555.

Llinás R, Volkind RA (1973). The olivocerebellar system:
functional properties as revealed by harmaline-induced
tremor. Exp Brain Res 18:69.

Palay SL, Chan-Palay V (1974). "Cerebellar Cortex. Cytology and Organization." Berlin: Springer.

Sotelo C, Palay SL (1971). Altered axons and axon terminals
in the lateral vestibular nucleus of the rat: possible
example of axonal remodeling. Lab Invest 25:653.

Zimmermann H(1979). Commentary: vesicle recycling and transmitter release. Neurosci 4:1773.

CONTRIBUTION OF METALLIC IMPREGNATION TO NEUROANATOMY

**Eleventh International Congress of Anatomy:
Glial and Neuronal Cell Biology, pages 281—290
© 1981 Alan R. Liss, Inc., 150 Fifth Avenue, New York, NY 10011**

NEOCORTICAL ENDEAVOR: BASIC NEURONAL ORGANIZATION IN THE CORTEX OF HEDGEHOG

F. Valverde and L. López-Mascaraque

Sección de Neuroanatomía Comparada
Instituto Cajal, CSIC
Madrid, Spain

Among the insectivores, the hedgehog (<u>Erinaceus euro-</u>
<u>paeus</u>) is regarded as one of the most direct modern descen-
dants of the primitive placentals (Romer, 1974). It has
retained, apparently with minor variations, some basic characteristics of its early ancestors so that it is a good
reference for the study of what might be considered a pro-
totype of neocortical organization and a valid, though not
unique, model on neocortical phylogenetic development. This
study was designed to unravel some cytoarchitectural and
morphological details in the hedgehog's neocortex with the
aim to define types of local circuit neurons that might already be present in this cortex, the form and distribution
of axonal plexuses in different neocortical layers and the
specificity vs the non-specificity of particular neuronal
representatives in relation to homologous types described
in other species. This analysis was carried out using the
Golgi method (Valverde, 1978) and Nissl and fiber stains in
a total number of 46 young and adult hedgehogs.

GROSS ANATOMY, REGIONAL PARCELLATION AND CYTOARCHITECTURE
OF THE NEOCORTICAL FIELD.

Adult hedgehogs with 600-800 g of body weight have
brains measuring 16-18 mm in rostrocaudal length of which
one-third is occupied by a large olfactory bulb placed at
the rostro-ventral end of each hemisphere. A large, and
relatively deep rhinal fissure (Fig. 1B,R) circumvents the
entire lateral surface of the brain. The fissure runs very
high delimiting a relatively narrow, slightly protruded

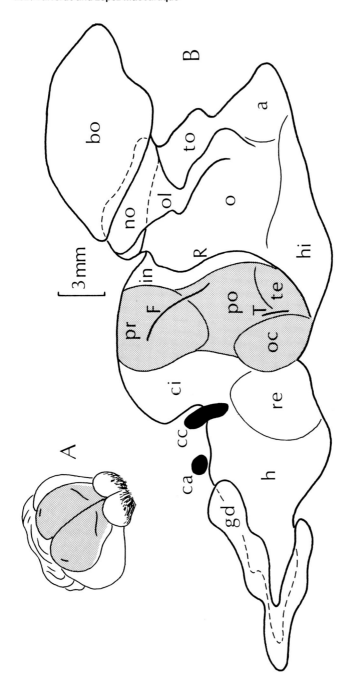

Figure 1. A. The brain of the hedgehog. B. Bidimensional map showing the different regions. The shaded areas correspond to the neocortex. (For abbreviations see text.)

neocortical field (Fig. 1, shaded area). Figure 1B shows a bidimensional representation of the entire cerebral mantle of the right hemisphere, reconstructed from measurements made with a curvimeter in serial, frontal, Nissl stained sections. The regional parcellation has been adapted from Brodmann (1909) and based on the works of Flores (1911) and Stephan (1956). In this map the neocortical field represents one-fifth of the entire surface of the brain, being slightly larger than the surface represented by the olfactory bulb; the remaining three-fifths of the cortical mantle corresponds to the very large archi- and paleo-cortices including associated transitional areas. A small rostrally placed corpus callosum is present (Fig. 1B, CC).

The regio praecentralis extends from the rostral pole to continue caudally with the regio postcentralis; the former is characterized by the great width of layer V and the low cell density; the latter is denser and more uniformly cellular. Caudally, the regio occipitalis shows slight cell condensation above layer V, indicating the presence of an internal granular layer (layer IV); laterally, a band of cortex relatively poor in radial fibers and a small shallow groove (Fig. 1B, T) separates it from the regio temporalis, as has been also noted by Hall and Diamond (1968).

The neocortex of the hedgehog is characterized by a poor cell lamination. Layer I is exceedingly thick; it measures 250-300 μm, and is formed by a large number of tangential bundles of myelinated fibers (Fig. 4A, F) and occasional large cells with axons ramifying here (Fig. 4A, a and 1a). This layer is permeated by a dense feltwork of spinous dendrites from underlying cells. Layer II forms a conspicuous cell band containing densely packed, polymorphic, large neurons. The darkly staining density of layer II throughout the neocortical field is the most distinguishing feature of the cortex; this characteristic was observed in a number of insectivores as a common, primitive, architectonic feature and aptly named "accentuated layer II" by Sanides and Sanides (1974). The cell bodies often aggregate into clumps containing several dozen densely packed neurons (Figs. 2A and 4A: cb). Under layer II there is a uniform band of cells composed of medium-sized pyramidal and polymorphic neurons arranged in short vertical rows. We interpret this band as layer III-IV, since a definite internal granular layer is never present except in the regio occipitalis where this stratum receives geniculo-cortical projections (Lende and

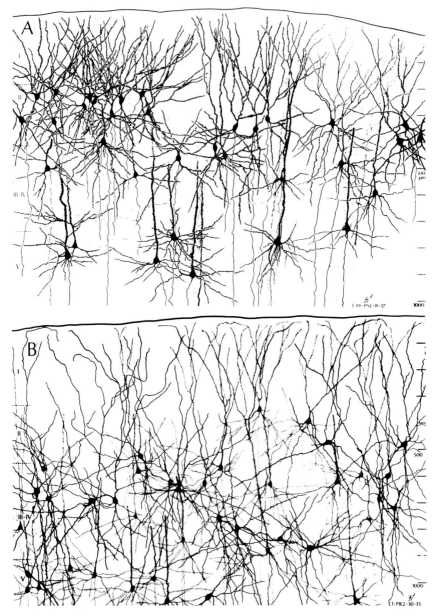

Figure 2. Transverse sections through the regio postcentralis. A: Large stellate cells with spinous dendrites and conventional pyramidal cells. B: Large stellate cells with smooth dendrites. Golgi method.

Sadler, 1967; Gould et al., 1978; Kaas et al., 1970). Layer
V contains large pyramidal cells (Fig. 2A: V) scattered
through light bands containing densely interwoven basal dendrites and collateral dendrites of apical shafts. Layer VI
is distinguished by the existence of horizontal rows of polymorphic and pyramidal cells separated by horizontal fascicles
of myelinated fibers detached out from the underlying white
matter. The total thickness of the neocortex varies from
800-1000 μm in the frontal regions to 600-800 μm in more
caudal fields.

In fiber and Golgi stained preparations we have found
the existence of numerous radial bundles of myelinated fibers,
predominating in the posterior half of the neocortex, as
shown earlier by Flores (1911). These radial bundles detach
from the white matter and ascend vertically to enter the lower
stratum of layer I where they run tangentially for variable
distances (Fig. 4A, F). At the present moment we can only
speculate that they might represent a strong zonal input of
unknown origin (thalamic, paleocortical).

THE BASIC NEURONAL COMPONENTS OF A PRIMITIVE NEOCORTEX

The study by the Golgi method of a large collection of
preparations from the neocortex of the hedgehog show the
presence of neuronal varieties which, on one hand, differs
from those found in common laboratory animals while, on the
other, they have surprising resemblances to neurons believed
to be specific for higher vertebrate brains. Some cell types
show features corresponding to primitive cortices: this is
the case of the stellate, spiny neurons of the accentuated
layer II that has been so thoroughly discussed by Sanides
(1970, 1974). Indeed, the Golgi image of a section through
the regio postcentralis in the adult hedgehog (Fig. 2A) shows
most clearly the predominance of such spiny, stellate cells;
they are provided with numerous spreading dendritic branches
entering the wide layer I (Fig. 4A: b). This cell is typical
of paleocortical formations: it resembles neurons found in
allocortex where a dense row of cell bodies stands out
clearly with notable external and internal dendritic spreads.
Typical pyramidal cells populate the underlying cortical
layers. This would suggest an overlapping of two types of
cortical formations: one consisting of large, spiny, stellate
cells with marked dendritic extensions toward a broad layer
I with strong fiber input, and a second type of cortex in

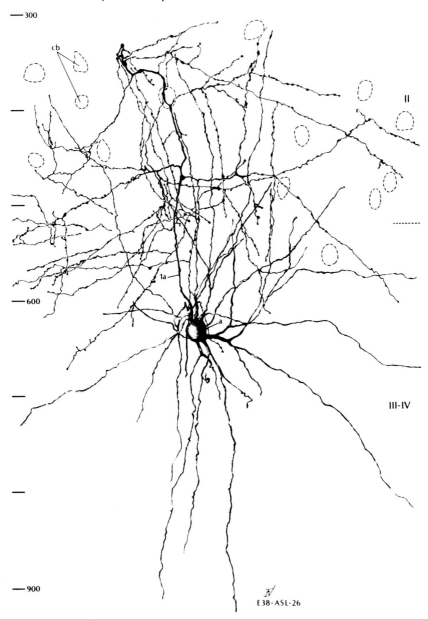

Figure 3. Large stellate cell with long and smooth dendrites and an ascending axon that branches mainly in layer II. This cell is typical in the neocortex of the hedgehog. Golgi method.

which pyramidal cells share with local circuit neurons a more elaborate type of architecture. The first type is very similar to that found in cortical olfactory centers.

Scattered through the midcortical layers and especially in layer III-IV we have found a type of large multipolar cell with smooth, very long dendrites and axons that extend for considerable distances (Fig. 3). This neuronal type has been found frequently in all neocortical regions; their dendrites are long and span through all cortical layers, while the axonal arborization seems to extend preferentially towards layer II. The very thick axonal trunk resolves into long and straight collaterals sometimes recurring toward the deep layers. Similar types of neurons have been found in the visual cortex of the mouse (Valverde and Ruiz-Marcos, 1969). Less frequently, we have been able to observe the existence of bipolar cells, stellate cells with spinous dendrites and local axons, and deep cells with ascending axons. However, these show a marked degree of unspecificity since they did not show any elaborate terminal axonal formations. In con- trast, specific neuronal varieties, as chandelier cells, were frequently observed (Fig. 4B, a); their axonal arboriza- tion formed bouton aggregates, vertically oriented, which made synapses with the initial segments of axons of pyramidal neurons (Fairén and Valverde, 1980). The inset in figure 4B shows a detailed drawing of the specific terminal portions (STPs). Similarly, the "axo-axonal" interneuron found by Somogyi (1977) in the visual cortex of the rat, effects the same type of contacts.

In conclusion, the study of the hedgehog's neocortex, at the level of resolution provided by the Golgi method, sug- gests a primitive stage of cortical evolution in which a paleocortical organization entirely covers a typical neo- cortical formation containing rather elaborate neuronal varieties.

REFERENCES

Brodmann K (1909). "Vergleichende Lokalisations-lehre der Grosshirnrinde." Leipzig: Johan Ambrosius Barth, p 194.
Fairén A, Valverde F (1980). A specialized type of neuron in the visual cortex of the cat. A Golgi and electron microscope study of chandelier cells. J Comp Neurol (in press).

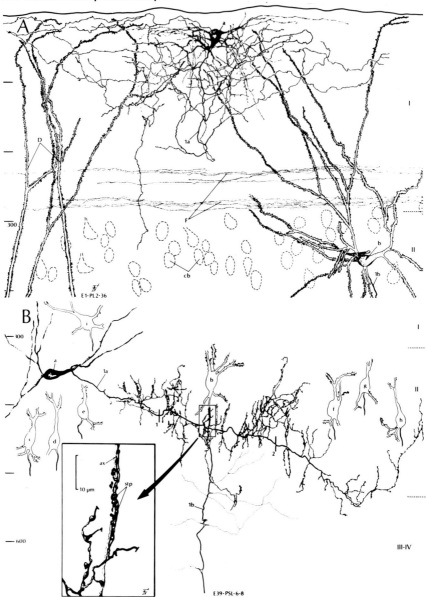

Figure 4. A: One cell in layer I with the axon branching in this layer. B: One example of a chandelier neuron in layer II with details of specific terminal portions around the axon of a large stellate cell. Golgi method.

Flores A (1911). Die Myeloarchitektonik und die Myelogenie des Cortex Cerebri beim Igel (Erinaceus europaeus). J Psychol Neurol 17:215.

Gould HJ, Hall WC, Ebner FF (1978). Connections of the visual cortex in the hedgehog (Paraechinus hypomelas). I. Thalamocortical projections. J Comp Neurol 177:445.

Hall WC, Diamond IT (1968). Organization and function of the visual cortex in the hedgehog: I. Cortical cytoarchitecture and thalamic retrograde degeneration. Brain Behav Evol 1:181.

Kaas J, Hall WC, Diamond IT (1970). Cortical visual areas I and II in the hedgehog: Relation between evoked potential maps and architecture subdivisions. J Neurophysiol 33:595.

Lende RA, Sadler KM (1967). Sensory and motor areas in neocortex of hedgehog (Erinaceus). Brain Res 5:390.

Romer AS (1974). "Vertebrate Paleontology." Chicago and and London: The University of Chicago Press, p 207.

Sanides F (1970). Functional architecture of motor and sensory cortices in primates in the light of a new concept of neocortex evolution. In Noback CR, Montagna W (eds): "Advances in Primatology Vol 1, The Primate Brain." New York: Appleton-Century-Crofts, p 137.

Sanides D, Sanides F (1974). A comparative Golgi study of the neocortex in insectivores and rodents. Z mikrosk anat Forsch 88:957.

Somogyi P (1977). A specific "axo-axonal" interneuron in the visual cortex of the rat. Brain Res 136:345.

Stephan H (1956). Vergleichend-anatomische Untersuchungen an Insektivorengehirnen. II. Oberflächermessungen am Allocortex im Hinblick auf funktionelle und phylogenetische Probleme. Morph Jb 97:123.

Valverde F (1978). The organization of area 18 in the monkey. Anat Embryol 154:305.

Valverde F, Ruiz-Marcos A (1969). Dendritic spines in the visual cortex of the mouse: Introduction to a mathematical model. Brain Res 8:269.

ABBREVIATIONS

a	Nucleus amygdaloideus	gd	Gyrus dentatus
bo	Bulbus olfactorius	h	Hippocampus
ca	Commissura anterior	hi	Regio hippocampica
cc	Corpus callosum	in	Regio insularis
ci	Regio cingularis	no	Nucleus olfactorius
F	Sulcus frontalis	o	Regio olfactoria

oc Regio occipitalis
ol Tractus olfactorius
po Regio postcentralis
pr Regio praecentralis
R Sulcus rhinalis

re Regio retrosplenialis
T Sulcus temporalis
te Regio temporalis
to Tuberculum olfactorium

Eleventh International Congress of Anatomy:
Glial and Neuronal Cell Biology, pages 291–301
© **1981 Alan R. Liss, Inc., 150 Fifth Avenue, New York, NY 10011**

THE GOLGI-EM PROCEDURE: A TOOL TO STUDY NEOCORTICAL
INTERNEURONS

A. Fairén, J. DeFelipe and R. Martínez-Ruiz

Sección de Neuroanatomía Comparada
Instituto Cajal, CSIC
Madrid 6, Spain

Knowledge of the basic intrinsic circuits operating in
the cerebral cortex must be based upon an exact understanding of the interneurons that contribute to them. Classifi-
cations have been based on a number of approaches, and indeed
the most used one has been the analysis of Golgi preparations. However, data from such analyses are difficult to
reconcile into a simple scheme. In order to establish a
basis for classification additional data are necessary,
especially on the afferent and efferent connectivity of the
local neurons.

Connectivity can be studied to advantage using the Golgi-
EM procedure, by which geometrical aspects revealed by the
Golgi stain can be correlated to the patterns of synaptic
connections observed in the electron microscope. In the
present report, the criteria that have led to identification of two particular types of interneurons in the cerebral
cortex will be discussed; furthermore, some technical conditions that improve suitability of a recently developed
Golgi-EM technique (Fairén et al., 1977) for the study of
local circuits in the cerebral cortex will be considered.
The technical principles set down here, however, may be of a
more general applicability.

TECHNICAL CONSIDERATIONS

Since in a previous report Fairen et al. (1977) described the procedures in detail, only certain novel technical aspects will be discussed here.

GOLGI-EM PROCEDURE

Golgi Staining and Gold Toning

In addition to the rapid Golgi impregnation recommended earlier, Golgi-Kopsch material (Colonnier, 1964) yields satisfactory ultrastructural preservation and has the important advantage of allowing for the use of E-PTA (Bloom and Aghajanian, 1968) as the electron "stain", so that the forms of the synapses in which the deimpregnated neurons participate are readily displayed.

After sectioning, the glycerinated Golgi material is examined in the light microscope to select suitable neurons for electron microscopy. This step is not trivial, since illumination of sections in the microscope stage seems to be an essential prerequisite for a successful toning. As pointed out by Blackstad (1980), white light reduces silver chromate into metallic silver. Thus, the mechanism of gold toning, of reduced silver preparations (Feigin and Naoumenko, 1976), would not differ essentially from that of Golgi impregnated sections. Illumination can be set up to facilitate bulk processing. We use a 150 W bulb, placed at a distance of some 10 cm from a petri dish containing the Golgi sections in glycerol. This kind of illumination raises the temperature appreciably, and care must be taken to keep the glycerol at 20°-25°C; however, at lower temperatures no optimal results are obtained. For each material, the appropriate times must be determined by trial, but it must be realized that they need to be rather long. This is especially true with regard to Golgi-Kopsch material.

By properly illuminating the sections prior to gold toning, a larger number of neurons are observed in the light microscope that maintain all their morphological features after deimpregnation. However, whereas a given illumination time can be adequate for the structures situated near the cut surfaces of the sections, the ones placed more deeply may remain refractory to gold toning; prolonging illumination times overcomes this difficulty.

Gold toning is effected with an ice cold, dilute aqueous solution of yellow gold chloride after the glycerol has been removed (Fairén et al., 1977). A procedure that improves control of the deposit of gold into the impregnated structures has been referred to elsewhere (Fairén and

Valverde, 1980). In brief, the method consists in immersing tissue sections in the gold chloride solution for repeated 5 minute periods and washing them in ice cold distilled water in the intervals. After each period of gold treatment a test section is taken out of the distilled water, treated by sodium thiosulfate and observed in the light microscope; in this way, the amount of toning reached can be followed. However, false conclusions can be drawn if test sections are observed after short times in sodium thiosulfate because these sections are illuminated and warmed during observation (Blackstad, 1980). Although it does not seem essential, oxalic acid treatment (using an ice cold 0.02% solution repeated in 5 minute periods) can be effected after toning is considered almost completed.

Once the process is finished, the tissue sections are washed in distilled water and deimpregnated in 1% sodium thiosulfate, as described before (Fairén et al., 1977).

Staining Golgi-Kopsch Sections for Electron Microscopy

For this purpose, two variations exist. One is to osmicate tissue, using a buffered 2% solution of osmic acid with 2% potassium dichromate added to avoid excessive darkening of the tissue. Staining is completed by "en bloc" uranyl acetate, the ultrathin sections being stained with lead citrate. The alternative is the E-PTA staining method of Bloom and Aghajanian (1968) that can be applied successfully to deimpregnated Golgi-Kopsch sections. To this end, the tissue sections are soaked in ethanolic phosphotungstic acid solution (Bloom and Aghajanian, 1968; D.G. Jones, 1973) for 12 hours, rinsed in absolute ethanol and embedded as usual. No staining of ultrathin sections is made. As an illustration, Fig. 1 shows several dendritic portions of a pyramidal cell in layer III of the visual cortex of the cat. Although in this preparation, membranes are not clearly discernible, gold particles define the boundaries of the labelled profiles quite accurately; mitochondria and microtubules appear faintly stained. In Fig. 1A, a synapse is seen contacting the shaft of a dendritic branch arising from the apical dendrite (Ap). In Fig. 1B, a similar synaptic complex on a dendritic shaft is apparent. In both cases, presynaptic dense projections and cleft material are visible; the postsynaptic band is shallow, so that both synapses correspond to the symmetrical type seen in conventionally stained material. In asymmetrical synapses (Fig. 1C), the band of postsynaptic

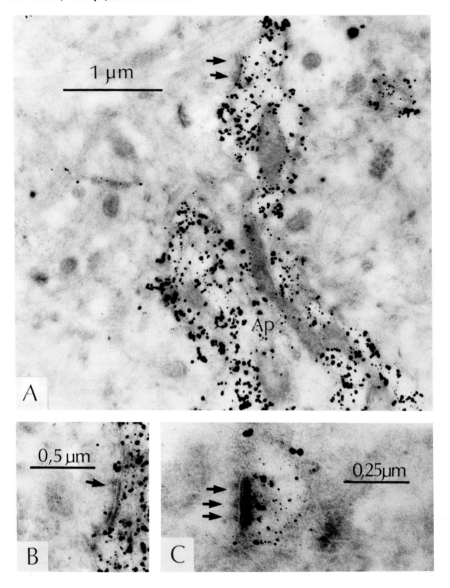

Figure 1. Golgi-Colonnier impregnation, E-PTA staining. Dendritic portions of a pyramidal cell from layer III of the visual cortex of the cat. Arrows point to dense projections. A and B: Symmetrical synapses on shafts of collateral dendrites. C: An asymmetrical synapse on a dendritic spine.

material is thicker.

By using this combined method, the mapping of afferent inputs converging upon definite neurons (Davis and Sterling, 1979; White, 1979) would be facilitated; synapses can be identified more easily because of the specifity of the stain. It can also be useful to trace extrinsic afferents, for, as shown by Sloper and Powell (1979), E-PTA also stains degenerating axon terminals.

Factors That Affect the Appearance and Distribution of Gold Particles

The size of gold particles at the ultrastructural level depends on illumination: the longer the illumination the smaller and more numerous the particles (Blackstad, 1980). Diffusion of gold particles around the originally impregnated structures is a somewhat annoying phenomenon leading to poor resolution; this undesired effect is substantially corrected in our material by proper exposure to light prior to gold toning. In addition, the presence of low concentrations of glycerol in the gold chloride solution during toning leads to some diffusion. It seems that small amounts of glycerol enhance photosensitivity of gold chloride solutions. Therefore, the glycerol should be carefully washed out from the sections and the gold toning done in subdued light. Finally, the use of oxalic acid in our procedure produces images of perikarya (and large dendrites) in which the gold particles are preferentially in a peripheral location; without oxalic acid they tend to distribute more evenly in the cytoplasm. At the light microscope level, however, oxalic acid improves contrast of the finest axonal branches.

LOCAL EFFERENT CONNECTIVITY: A BASIS FOR TYPING OF CORTICAL INTERNEURONS

Since limitations of space preclude us from entering into a detailed discussion, only two types of interneurons will be considered in which certain properties of their local axonal arborizations have served as distinctive criteria for classification.

The first type to be examined is the chandelier cell,

the subject of several Golgi-EM studies (Somogyi, 1977, 1979; Somogyi et al., 1979; Fairén and Valverde, 1980). Its axonal arborization is most characteristic: recurrent branches from the primary axonal stem form outstanding vertical rows of boutons (specific terminal portions or STPs). These make symmetrical synaptic contacts only with initial axon segments of pyramidal cells (Figs. 2 and 3); this kind of specificity is a unique feature of this type of interneuron and contrasts with the efferent synaptic patterns displayed by other types.

Fig. 2A depicts several boutons (labelled 1 to 11) surrounding the initial segment of a pyramidal neuron from layer III of the visual cortex of the cat. They were identified in the light microscope as belonging to a STP from a chandelier cell. This preparation is from material impregnated by the Golgi-Colonnier procedure, deimpregnated and stained with E-PTA, and shows up membranes relatively well, as is frequently observed in this type of material. The distinctive features of the initial segment are visible. E-PTA staining reveals the axoaxonic synapses clearly (Fig. 2B, arrowheads); in Fig. 2C, a higher magnification of such a synapse reveals the intrasynaptic line and a thin postsynaptic band, whereas dense projections are somewhat obscured by the gold particles. Gold toned rapid Golgi preparations are also suitable to show synaptic contracts between STPs and initial axon segments. As an illustration, the initial segment of a pyramidal cell from layer II-III of the visual cortex of the mouse is shown in Fig. 3. (See also, Fairén and Valverde, 1980).

Chandelier cells have been found in a number of species. Valverde and López-Mascaraque (this volume) have presented light microscopical evidence that a similar cell exists in the neocortex of hedgehogs. Comparison between Figs. 2 and 3 illustrates how the number of boutons that contact each initial segment, derived from one STP, is higher in cats than in mice. Correspondingly, Golgi preparations reveal more elaborate STPs in higher species. It seems that this fact reflects an evolutive trend, as suggested previously (Fairén and Valverde, 1980).

Figure 2 A: Cat visual cortex. Golgi-Colonnier, E-PTA staining. Synaptic boutons (labelled from 1 to 11) from a terminal portion of a chandelier cell surrounding the axon initial segment of a pyramidal cell. B and C: are higher magnifications of boutons 1 to 3 in an adjacent section.

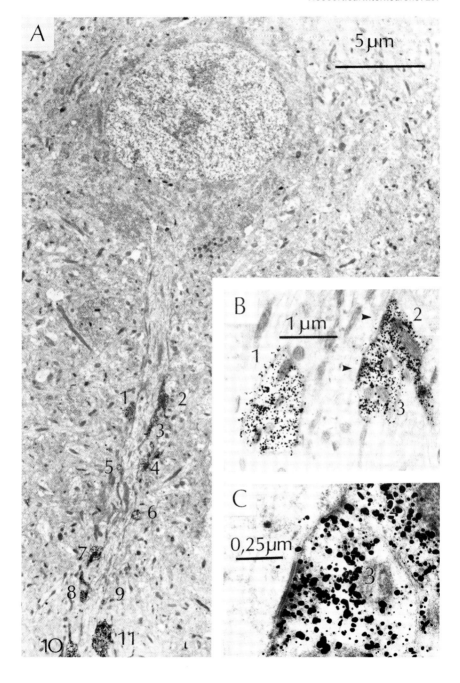

A 5 μm

B 1 μm

C 0,25 μm

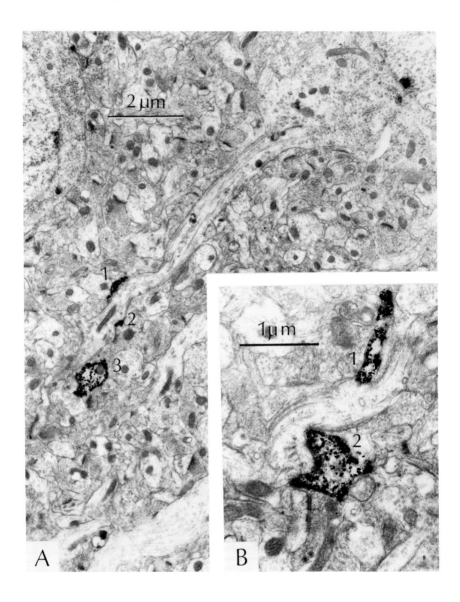

Figure 3. A: Rapid Golgi method. Boutons (1 to 3) from a terminal portion of a chandelier cell in area 41 contacting a pyramidal cell from layer II-III. B: Higher magnification of boutons 1 and 2 in adjacent section.

A second type of interneuron displays also a distinctive though less conspicuous image of the axonal tree. In rats the primary axonal trunk is usually ascending and gives rise to secondary branches that form arcades; tertiary branches are oblique or horizontal and are studied with dilatations. These dilatations engage in symmetrical synaptic contracts with a variety of different postsynaptic elements (Peters and Fairén, 1978; Peters and Proskauer, 1980). Interneurons displaying a similar axon geometry are common in diverse species (e.g., type 2 interneurons: E.G. Jones, 1975) and are also present in the hedgehog neocortex (Valverde and López-Mascaraque, this Symposium). Given the similarity of their axonal plexuses it would not seem too adventurous to predict that all these cells would produce an identical pattern of efferent contracts; this must be based, however, on direct observations of similar neurons in several species. Our preliminary observations in the cat visual cortex reveal a similar morphology of the axonal plexuses, although some tertiary branches are vertical. The electron microscope reveals a pattern of synaptic connections effected by these axons in the neocortex of the cat which is consistent with that previously found in rats.

In conclusion, although it is evident that other morphological criteria must not be disregarded, the examples chosen show that correlating the geometrical aspects of local axonal arborizations to the patterns of synaptic connections may serve to bring out important features of the intracortical circuits.

ACKNOWLEDGEMENTS

We wish to express our sincere gratitude to Prof. T.W. Blackstad, for allowing us access to his unpublished material. This work has been supported by a grant from Fundación E. Rodríguez Pascual.

REFERENCES

Blackstad TW (1980). Tract tracing by electron microscopy of Golgi preparations. In Heimer L, Robards, MJ (eds): "Neuroanatomical Tract Tracing Methods", New York: Plenum Press (in press).

Bloom FE, Aghajanian GF (1968). Fine structural and cytochemical analysis of the staining of synaptic junctions
with phosphotungstic acid. J. Ultrastr Res 22:361.
Colonnier M (1964). The tangential organization of the visual cortex. J Anat (Lond) 98:327.
Davis TL, Sterling P (1979). Microcircuitry of cat visual
cortex: classification of neurons in layer IV of area 17,
and identification of the patterns of lateral geniculate
input. J Comp Neur 188:599.
Fairén A, Peters A, Saldanha J (1977). A new procedure
for examining Golgi impregnated neurons by light and electron microscopy. J Neurocytol 6:311.
Fairén A, Valverde F (1980). A specialized type of neuron in
the visual cortex of cat. A Golgi and electron microscope
study of chandelier cells. J Comp Neur, in press.
Feigin I, Naoumenko J (1976). Some chemical principles
applicable to some silver and gold staining methods for
neuropathological studies. J Neuropath Exp Neur 35:495.
Jones DG (1973). Some factors affecting the PTA staining of
synaptic junctions. Z Zellforsch 143:301.
Jones EG (1975). Varieties and distribution of non-pyramidal
cells in the somatic sensory cortex of the squirrel monkey.
J Comp Neur 160:205.
Peters A, Fairén A (1978). Smooth and sparsely-spined stellate cells in the visual cortex of the rat: a study using
a combined Golgi-electron microscope technique. J Comp
Neur 181:129.
Peters A, Proskauer CC (1980). Synaptic relationships between
a multipolar stellate cell and a pyramidal neuron in the
rat visual cortex. A combined Golgi-electron microscope
study. J Neurocytol 9:163.
Sloper JJ, Powell TPS (1979). An experimental electron microscopic study of afferent connections to the primate motor
and somatic sensory cortices. Phil Trans R Soc Lond B
285:199.
Somogyi P (1977). A specific "axo-axonal" interneuron in the
visual cortex of the rat. Brain Res 136:345.
Somogyi P (1979). An interneurone making synapses specifically on the axon initial segment of pyramidal cells in the
cerebral cortex of the cat. J Physiol (Lond) 296:18P.
Somogyi P, Hodgson AJ, Smith AD (1979). An approach to tracing neuron networks in the cerebral cortex and basal
ganglia. Combination of Golgi staining, retrograde transport of horseradish peroxidase and anterograde degeneration
of synaptic boutons in the same material. Neuroscience 4:
1805.

White EL (1979).   Thalamocortical synaptic relations: a review with emphasis on the projections of specific thalamic nuclei to the primary sensory areas of the neocortex. Brain Res Rev 1:275.

Eleventh International Congress of Anatomy:
Glial and Neuronal Cell Biology, pages 303—310
© 1981 Alan R. Liss, Inc., 150 Fifth Avenue, New York, NY 10011

ELECTRON MICROSCOPY OF GOLGI IMPREGNATED NEURONS IN CAT
VISUAL CORTEX USED TO TRACE THALAMO-CORTICAL PROJECTIONS.

L.J. GAREY and J.P. HORNUNG

Institute of Anatomy, University of Lausanne,
Rue du Bugnon 9, 1011 Lausanne, Switzerland.

INTRODUCTION

Neurons of the lateral geniculate nucleus (LGN) of
the cat send axons to the visual cortex (VC) where they
terminate mainly in layer IV. It has been shown by electron microscopic study after LGN lesions that about 80% of
the thalamo-cortical axons terminate on dendritic spines
and the rest on dendritic shafts or neuronal somata (Colonnier and Rossignol, 1969; Garey and Powell, 1971).
However, only a small proportion of the neurons postsynaptic to thalamo-cortical axons can be identified in
standard electron micrographs. This is because, although
neuronal somata have ultrastructural features which are,
in general, specific for pyramidal or stellate cells
(Colonnier, 1968; Garey, 1971), dendrites (and even more
particularly spines) are difficult, if not impossible, to
attribute to either class of cortical cell. We know that
all thalamo-cortical axons probably end at synapses of the
asymmetrical variety and that only stellate cells seem to
receive asymmetrical axo-somatic synapses. However, both
stellate and pyramidal dendritic shafts can receive both
asymmetrical and symmetrical synapses, although the proportion of asymmetrical synapses is higher on stellate
dendrites. Furthermore, as spines of both neuronal types
are found in layer IV, it is not possible to decide which
spines receive fibres from the LGN, unless the cell is
marked in a way which can be used to distinguish stellates
from pyramids.

Such a marking technique exists at the light micro-scopic level: the Golgi method. However, the adaptation of this technique to electron microscopy had proved difficult and only since the gold-toning modification of Fairén, Peters and Saldanha (1977) became available has it been possible to combine light and electron microscopy of Golgi impregnated cells efficiently.

MATERIALS AND METHODS

Experiments were performed on adult cats anaesthe-tized with Nembutal. Stereotaxic lesions were made in the LGN of both hemispheres. After survivals of 3 to 4 days the animals were perfused with buffered paraformaldehyde and glutaraldehyde. After brief post-fixation, blocks of VC were removed and impregnated with the rapid Golgi tech-nique (Valverde, 1970). Blocks were stored in glycerol at 4°C and later sectioned at 100 µm on a sliding microtome, enclosed in a paraffin block to stabilize the tissue. Well impregnated neurons in area 17 of the VC were selected by light microscopy, excised from the sections and toned with gold chloride. The silver Golgi precipitate was then removed by treatment with sodium thiosulphate (Fairén et al., 1977). The selected neurons were still visible by light microscopy in the excised fragments which were then osmificated, stained with uranyl acetate, dehydrated and embedded in flat resin discs. Careful trimming and removal of 1 µm thick sections allowed the neuron to be approached for ultrathin sectioning. Series of up to 120 serial ultrathin sections were collected on single-slot grids coated with Formvar.

RESULTS

Several neurons in area 17 fulfilled the criteria of being classifiable by light microscopy, of good ultra-structural quality and contacted by degenerating termi-nals. Both pyramidal and stellate neurons proved to be targets for thalamo-cortical axons.

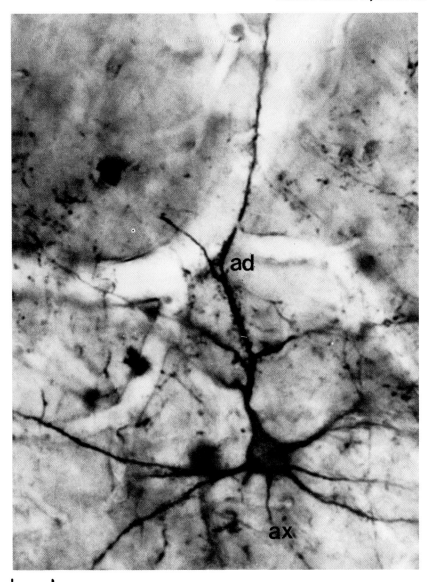

Fig. 1. Gold-toned Golgi preparation of pyramidal neuron in layer III of cat area 17. Note the spine-rich apical (ad) and basal dendrites and the axon initial segment (ax). Scale = 20 µm.

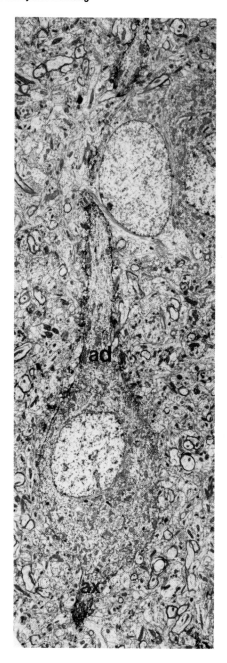

Fig. 2. Electron micrograph of the same neuron as in Fig. 1. The Golgi marking is clearly visible in the soma, apical dendrite (ad) and axon (ax). Scale = 3 μm.

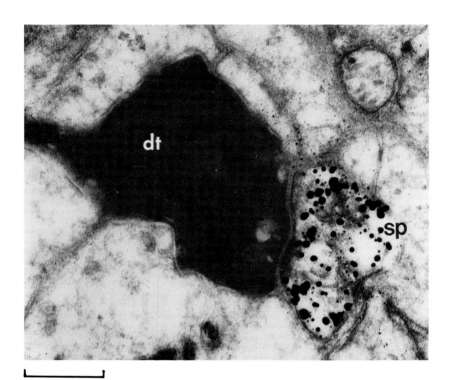

Fig. 3. Degenerating thalamo-cortical terminal (dt) on a marked spine (sp) of a basal dendrite of the neuron in Figs. 1 and 2.   Scale = 0.5 μm.

Pyramidal neurons were identified by their thick apical dendrite and five or so basal dendrites (Fig.1). All dendrites bore large numbers of spines. The axon left the lower border of the soma, which was either in layer III or V. Ultrastructurally (Fig. 2), pyramids received few axo-somatic synapses, and never asymmetrical ones. Their dendritic shafts also had few synapses, mainly symmetrical, but with rare asymmetrical examples. Spines received almost exclusively asymmetrical contacts.

Degenerating thalamo-cortical synapses manifested typical dark degneration reactions (Colonnier, 1964) and were always, when positively identifiable, of the asymmetrical variety (Fig. 3). Degenerating terminals were identified on spines of apical dendrites of layer III and V pyramids, and on spines of layer III pyramidal basal dendrites, in all cases as the dendrites ramified in layer IV or the lower part of layer III. In addition basal dendritic shafts of layer III pyramids received thalamo-cortical input.

Non-pyramidal neurons in layer IV were also targets for thalamic axons. These cells were either typically "stellate", with several radially arranged dendrites, or more bipolar, with the dendrites organized in two tufts. The dendrites were either spiny, although less so than pyramidal cells, or spine-free. Ultrastructurally, the spiny stellates could be distinguished from pyramids chiefly by the greater number of axo-somatic synapses, some of which were asymmetrical. The spine-free stellates were even more clearly different, in that they had yet more somatic contacts with a high proportion of asymmetrical; also, the dendritic shafts received many asymmetrical synapses. Thalamic terminals were identified innervating dendrites, somata and spines of stellate neurons, including all the types morphologically distinguishable.

DISCUSSION

The use of electron microscopy of Golgi impregnated cells has enabled the VC neurons post-synaptic to thalamo-cortical axons in cat to be identified. We have shown that both pyramidal and stellate neurons receive direct thalamo-cortical input, and that dendritic shafts and spines of both types are involved. It is already known that stellate somata also receive thalamic afferents (Colonnier and Rossignol, 1969; Garey and Powell, 1971). Thus it can be said that every neuronal surface known to be contacted by asymmetrical synapses in the layers receiving thalamic afferents is a potential candidate for such thalamic input. These findings in cat agree with those using similar techniques in rodents, both in visual and somatosensory cortex (Somogyi, 1978; White, 1978; Peters, Proskauer, Feldman and Kimerer, 1979).

The Golgi electron microscopic method has, then, enabled us to investigate cortical circuitry in more detail than previously, but it cannot give information as to the possible efferent pathways originating from the thalamically innervated neurons. However, other light microscopic techniques adapted for electron microscopy can help. For example, the use of horseradish peroxidase has enabled us to show that one type of stellate cell (the large spiny type) which is monosynaptically activated from the LGN, projects to the VC of the contralateral hemisphere by the corpus callosum (Hornung and Garey, 1980). More work is needed to further classify the identifiable cortical neurons according to their afferent and efferent connexions.

REFERENCES

Colonnier M (1964). Experimental degeneration in the cerebral cortex. J Anat (Lond) 98:47.

Colonnier M (1968). Synaptic patterns on different cell types in the different laminae of the cat visual cortex. An electron microscope study. Brain Research 9:268.

Colonnier M, Rossignol S (1969). Heterogeneity of the cerebral cortex. In Jasper HH, Ward AA, Pope A (eds): "Brain Mechanisms of the Epilepsies". Boston: Little, Brown, p 29.

Fairén A, Peters A, Saldanha J (1977). A new procedure for examining Golgi impregnated neurons by light and electron microscopy. J Neurocytology 6:311.

Garey LJ (1971). A light and electron microscopic study of the visual cortex of the cat and monkey. Proc Roy Soc Lond B 179:21.

Garey LJ, Powell, TPS (1971) An experimental study of the termination of the lateral geniculo-cortical pathway in the cat and monkey. Proc Roy Soc Lond B 179:41.

Hornung JP, Garey LJ (1980). A direct pathway from thalamus to visual callosal neurons in cat. Exper Brain Research 38:121.

Peters A, Proskauer C, Feldman M, Kimerer L (1979). The projection of the lateral geniculate nucleus to area 17 of the rat cerebral cortex. V. Degenerating axon terminals synapsing with Golgi impregnated neurons. J Neurocytology 8:331.

Somogyi P (1978). The study of Golgi stained cells and of experimental degeneration under the electron microscope: a direct method for the identification in the visual cortex of three successive links in a neuron chain. Neuroscience 3:167.

Valverde F (1970). The Golgi method. A tool for comparative structural analyses. In Nauta WJH, Ebbesson SOE (eds): "Contemporary Research Methods in Neuroanatomy", New York: Springer, p. 11.

White EL (1978). Identified neurons in mouse Sml cortex which are postsynaptic to thalamocortical axon terminals: a combined Golgi-electron micrsocopic and degeneration study. J Comp Neurol 181:627.

ACKNOWLEDGEMENTS

This work was supported by the Swiss National Science Foundation 3.0950.77.

Eleventh International Congress of Anatomy:
Glial and Neuronal Cell Biology, pages 311–317
© 1981 Alan R. Liss, Inc., 150 Fifth Avenue, New York, NY 10011

THE GOLGI METHODS AND THE ABNORMAL CEREBRAL
CORTEX: EPILEPSY AND AGING

Arnold B. Scheibel, M.D.

Departments of Anatomy and Psychiatry
and Brain Research Institute
UCLA Medical Center, Los Angeles, CA
U.S.A.

"Everyman, I will go with thee, and be thy
guide, in thy most need to go by thy side."

No technique in the lexicon of light microscopy exhibits the power and versatility of the
Golgi heavy metal impregnation methods. Its
capacity to make visible all portions of the
neuron together with its accompanying retinue of
neuroglia and vascular stroma remains unsur-
passed, even in a day of orthodromic and anti-
dromic axonal tracing and visualization, receptor labelling, and histological localization of
metabolically active components. Its time of
initial activity, during the forty years brack-
eting the turn of the century, was terminated
only when the information it produced had far
outdistanced correlatable physiological data.
Its renaissance in the early fifties and its
vigorous return in succeeding decades is trib-
ute not only to its own undiminished power but
to the vigor of the many other neuroscientific
methodologies which depend on - or are measured
against - the Golgi techniques.

It is, accordingly, somewhat strange that
this method was not applied to pathological
brain tissue until quite recently. Several
exceptions can be cited; primarily the studies
of De Moor (1898) calling attention to the loss
of dendritic spines (initially described by

Cajal in 1891) in human epileptic cortical
tissue, and the report of Monti (1895), demonstrating the loss of dendritic spines and development of dendritic nodules following severe
nutritional deficiency. The recent study by
Westrum et al. (1964) in which Golgi-Cox techniques were used to evaluate the pathology associated with experimental epilepsy in monkey and
the initial report by Marin-Padilla on cortical
fine structure in Patou Syndrome (1972) virtually
complete the roster. We (Scheibel and Scheibel,
unpubl.) had used Golgi methodology in examining
tissue blocks removed at surgery from four patients with temporal lobe epilepsy in 1952-1953,
but were too uncertain of the significance of the
results to report our findings. It is worth
noting that the Golgi was to us, at that time, a
"new technique", and there were initially no
other investigators (with the possible exception
of Clement Fox in Milwaukee) to whom we could
show our results or request confirmation.

We were given the opportunity to resume work
on this problem in 1969, receiving surgically
resected blocks of temporal lobe tissue removed
by Dr. Paul Crandall from patients with intractable uncal fits or seizure equivalents, at UCLA.
Study of a series of eleven patients (Scheibel,
Crandall and Scheibel, 1974) revealed a sequence
of dendritic changes in the hippocampal-dentate
complex of the majority of these patients. A
remarkable range of structural variations was
noted ranging from isolated patches of dendrite
spine loss associated with dendritic nodulation
on a portion of a dendrite to massively denuded
dendrite shafts with increasingly bizarre distortions and swellings. In many instances, these
changes appeared to progress toward dendrite
fragmentation and loss, culminating in cell death
and reactive gliosis. We were particularly
interested by the wide range of cell dendrite
changes, from the isolated, highly localized
"string of pearls" deformity of a single dendrite tip, to widespread spine loss, dendrite
deformation and cell death. Even in the dentate
fascia, apparently more resistant to such massive
tissue destructive changes, the dendrite ensem-
bles showed dramatic conformational changes such

as collapse inward upon the central axis of the arbor (the closed parasol deformity) and widespread in-unison bending of dendrite shaft systems toward one side, like a field of wheat before the wind (the windblown look). The significance of such changes has not been clarified but we assume that the distortions arise in response, at lease in the latter case, to adjacent areas of gliosis and cicatrization, "pulling" the dendrite shafts toward the more disturbed sites.

The spontaneous seizures of certain strains of Mongolian Gerbils provide a useful natural model of the human ictal state. Ongoing Golgi studies (Paul et al., 1979) have identified significant differences in dendritic spine density on hippocampal pyramidal cells between seized and non-seized animals. Examination of Golgi material also suggested differences in the presynaptic terminals impinging on these dendrite systems. Correlated examination of such terminals (mossy tufts) with the electron microscope has confirmed and extended these impressions. Golgi methods have thus been able to reveal, for the first time, evidence of both pre- and postsynaptic structural change related to the epileptic state.

An ever broader range of histological changes is revealed by Golgi analysis of tissue from aged, senescent, and/or demented patients. Despite the ever-present threat of postmortem artifact which must be faced in tissue removed from the human brain six, twelve, or even eighteen hours after death, a great deal of information can be gleaned from such material. Two factors which appear to make this possible are the apparently greater resistance of brain tissue from the aged to autolysis, and the 'forgiving' nature of the Golgi techniques, especially when contrasted with the demands of electron microscopy. Using the cerebral neocortex as model, the most frequently noted sequence of changes includes patchy spine loss and irregular swelling of cell body and proximal dendrite shaft, leading to a characteristic 'lumpy' silhouette. Horizontally oriented dendrite

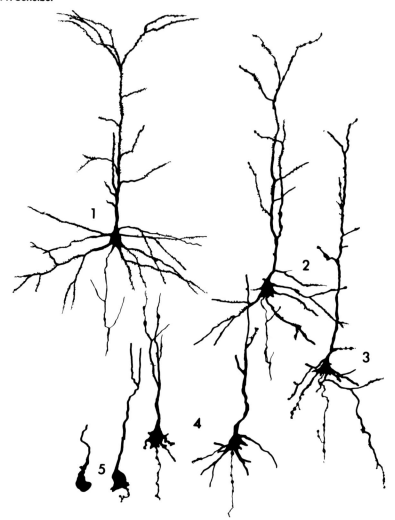

Figure 1   Sequence of changes in large cortical
pyramidal neurons in human neocortex. Starting
with the mature, intact neuron at 1, dendritic
spines are lost over increasing areas of dendrite
membrane, as the dendrite shafts become lumpy
and nodulated (2 and 3). There is progressive
loss of the basilar dendrite system (3, 4, and 5)
resulting in irregular, swollen somata bearing
rudimentary apical shafts which finally disappear
as the neurons die (5). Based on Golgi stained
sections from the superior temporal lobe of
patients of varying ages.

systems are selectively lost, including the
oblique branches of the apical shaft and, most
noticeably, the basilar dendrite systems. It is
interesting that these dendrites are also the
last to mature during development. Final stages
of histopathological change include fragmentation
of the apical shaft, pyknosis of the cell body,
and reactive growth of fibrillary astrocytes (Fig. 1).

Most of these changes have been followed in
pyramidal cells of layers 3 and 5 in the association areas, primarily superior and middle
frontal gyri, and the parieto-temporal zone. It
has been more difficult to draw conclusions about
the often-more-difficult-to-stain stellate or
local circuit cells. We have found, much to our
surprise, that the giant pyramidal cells of Betz
of the motor cortex and the large pyramidal
cells of Meynert in the visual cortex seem especially vulnerable to the aging process. Using the
Betz cell as model (Scheibel, Tomiyasu and
Scheibel, 1977), changes are frequently noted
in neurologically normal patients as early as
the fourth decade of life, and 70-80% of the total complement of Betz pyramids may be lost by the
seventh decade of life. In the cat (Kaplan and
Scheibel, unpubl.), large Betz and Meynert cells
show spine loss as early as the second to third
year of life, suggesting that this precocious
series of histological events is not species-
specific. Work is continuing in an effort to
evaluate the meaning of these early changes in
the largest cortical pyramids.

whatever the course of these specific
patterns of vulnerability, there are several
thinkable consequences of selective attrition
of Betz pyramids. As we have indicated in previous studies (1977), the specific inhibitory
function of these neurons on large extensor
(anti-gravity) muscles and their subsidiary role
in facilitation of apposed flexor systems gives
them a critical role in unloading weight-bearing
joints just before inception of a patterned
motor act. Their widespread loss inevitably
removes this initial lysis of anti-gravity tone,
causing motor activity to occur against a background of enhanced resistance. This is believed

likely to lead to the "slowing down," increasing stiffness, and discomfort in the lower extremities, of which so many older individuals complain.

Today the methods of Golgi are increasingly in demand, defining changes in morphology and connectivity in a wide range of dementing diseases, in neurological syndromes and even in certain types of severe psychiatric illness. One may recall the comment of an unnamed neuroanatomist at the end of the last century who, wondering at the broad application of Golgi methodology throughout brain research, is reported to have said, "Next they will Golgify potatoes." For us, the endless vigor of the method might well be epitomized in its final application to the problem of schizophrenia (Scheibel and Kovelman, unpubl.).

REFERENCES

De Moor J (1898). La mécanisme et le signification de l'état moniliforme des neurons. Ann Soc Sci Bruxelles Ser 2 7:205.

Marin-Padilla M (1972). Structural abnormalities of the cerebral cortex in human chromosomal aberrations. A Golgi study. Brain Res 44:625.

Monti A (1895). Sur les altérations du système nerveux dans l'inanition. Arch Ital Biol 24:347

Paul L, Fried I, Watanabe K, Scheibel A (1979). On structural substrates of epileptic behavior in the Mongolian Gerbil. Soc Neurosci Abstr 5:195.

Ramon y Cajal S (1911). "Histologie du Système Nerveux de l'Hommes et des Vertébrés." Paris: Maloine, 2 Vol.

Scheibel ME, Crandall P, Scheibel AB (1974). The hippocampaldentate complex in temporal lobe epilepsy. Epilepsia 15:55.

Scheibel ME, Lindsay RD, Tomiyasu U, Scheibel AB (1975). Progressive dendritic changes in aging human cortex. Exp Neurol 47:392

Scheibel ME, Tomiyasu U, Scheibel AB (1977). The aging human Betz cell. Exp Neurol 56:598

Westrum L, White L, Ward A (1964). Morphology of the experimental epileptic focus. J Neurosurg 21:1033.

DEVELOPMENT OF THE BRAIN

Eleventh International Congress of Anatomy:
Glial and Neuronal Cell Biology, pages 321 – 329
© **1981 Alan R. Liss, Inc., 150 Fifth Avenue, New York, NY 10011**

RECENT ADVANCES IN CHILD GROWTH AND DEVELOPMENT

Alex F. Roche

Fels Research Institute, Department of Pediatrics
Wright State University School of Medicine
Yellow Springs, Ohio, U.S.A.

THE ADIPOCYTE NUMBER HYPOTHESIS

The adipocyte number hypothesis states obesity during infancy is associated with an excessive increase in the number of adipocytes and that, as a result, there is an increased number of such cells throughout life, making such individuals prone to obesity at all ages (Hirsch & Knittle 1970). To evaluate this hypothesis it is necessary to consider briefly the methods by which adipocyte number and size are determined. The number of adipocytes is calculated from estimates of total body fat and of adipocyte mean size. Errors are involved in the determination of total body fat, and adipocyte size varies with the site examined or even among small areas within sites (Gurr & Kirtland 1978). Furthermore, in human beings it is impossible to identify empty adipocytes (Widdowson & Shaw 1973). Nevertheless, there is considerable agreement that the obese have increased numbers of adipocytes containing fat and that weight reduction is associated with a diminution in the size but not the number of these cells (Björntorp & Sjöström 1971).

It has been claimed that the later the stated age of onset of obesity, the larger the adipocytes (Apfelbaum, Brigant & Duret 1973). The inference is that obesity that begins when the number of adipocytes is increasing is associated with an increased number of adipocytes whereas obesity developing later is associated with an enlargement of existing adipocytes. Contrary findings indicate that the major determinant of the number of adipocytes is the amount of adipose tissue (Häger 1977).

The newly born infant has about one-fortieth as many adipocytes containing fat as the adult (Brook 1972). The increase in number is slight during the first year of life; most of the increase in total body fat during this period is due to hypertrophy of adipocytes which is not in agreement with the adipocyte number hypothesis (Häger et al. 1977). In adulthood the number of adipocytes containing fat is fairly stable even if there are large changes in the amount of body fat (Salans et al. 1971), but experimental obesity in adult rats is associated with an increase in the number of adipocytes (Lemonnier 1972).

Cross-sectional studies indicate adipocytes enlarge in normal children until 4 years; then their size remains fairly constant to 12 years but it increases during pubescence and adolescence (Hirsch & Knittle 1970). Others have reported rapid increases in adipocyte size from birth to 1 year but little change from then to adulthood (Häger et al. 1977). Serial data show the number of adipocytes increases until at least 16 years and that changes in estimated total body fat during pubescence are correlated positively and approximately equally with changes in either adipocyte number or adipocyte size (Roche, Chumlea, Siervogel, Knittle & Webb, unpublished data).

Serial Data

The adipocyte number hypothesis provided a cellular basis for the claim that obese infants tend to become obese adults. Few substantive reports concern the long-term natural history of subcutaneous adipose tissue or other indices of obesity. Almost all reported studies are based on recall or hospital records of doubtful relevance and accuracy. Findings from the most prominent studies do not support the notion that obese infants are predestined to become obese adults. Hernesniemi, Zachmann and Prader (1974) reported very low coefficients between subcutaneous fat thicknesses at four sites at the ages of 10 months and 15 years. Data from the major longitudinal studies in the United States for large samples, using many sites, show low correlations between subcutaneous fat thicknesses in infancy, measured as skinfolds or on radiographs, and the corresponding measures at 16 years (Roche, Chumlea, Eichorn, Himes, McCammon, Reed, Siervogel & Valadian, unpublished data). Wachholder (1976) reported very low correlations between subcutaneous fat thicknesses during

infancy and those at inflections during the pubescent spurt
in stature.

The percentage of body fat is greater than average in
children who recover from marasmus or kwashiorkor (Ashworth
1969). Also, there is no evidence that an increased number
of adipocytes predisposes to obesity. In summary, it must
be concluded that the hypothesis lacks convincing support.
Nevertheless, the work generated by the hypothesis has added
important new dimensions to our still incomplete understanding of the natural history of obesity.

POSSIBLE CATCH-UP GROWTH IN THE BRAIN

Some factors retard brain growth and development but it
is not clear whether this retardation is reversible. It is
difficult to interpret the early work in this area relating
to malnourished children because their nutritional and social
rehabilitation was incomplete. The general conclusion from
such studies that catch-up growth of the brain occurs only
if there is intervention before the age of 1 year may need
revision.

"Catch-up" growth is an acceleration during which growth
is more rapid than usual for age and sex. This acceleration
must occur in an individual who was retarded in growth immediately before the acceleration. The recognition of catch-
up growth in the brain depends, therefore, on knowledge of
the timing and rates of brain growth in normal children. The
significance of catch-up growth depends on the associated
microscopic and biochemical changes in the brain and on
function in affected children.

Brain Development and Growth in Normal Children

The morphological changes during brain development and
growth include: cell division and migration, enlargement of
neurones, growth of axons and dendrites in specific directions, formation of synapses, proliferation of glial cells,
and myelination. The timing and the extent of these processes differ among brain regions as does the development of
enzymes. Interference with the fixed sequence of morphological and biochemical events during the growth and maturation
of the brain may be irreversible (Winick, Brasel & Rosso

1972). In other words, if a process does not occur at the
normal time there will be a permanent functional deficit.
It has been hypothesized that the development and growth of
the brain are vulnerable to permanent restriction if a dele-
terious factor operates during periods of rapid change (Dobbing 1968). This concept denies the possibility of catch-
up growth.

The total number of cells in the brain can be determined
from the total DNA content of the brain. Mean cell size is
estimated by dividing total brain protein by the number of
cells on the assumption that all brain protein is intracellular. These methods do not distinguish between various
types of brain cells.

Malnutrition, during the period when brain cells divide
rapidly, reduces the rate of this division, leading to fewer
brain cells than normal; this deficit is said to be permanent. When brain cells cease to divide, they continue to
enlarge. Malnutrition during this phase limits this enlargement or causes a reduction in size but these effects are reversible. Malnutrition after brain growth is complete has
little or no effect on either cell size or number (Winick &
Noble 1966).

The small spurt in the number of brain cells from 10 to
18 weeks of gestation is probably due to an increase in the
number of neurones (Dobbing & Sands 1970). During this spurt
the brain is invulnerable to nutritional insults but can be
affected by irradiation, virus infections, and chromosomal
abnormalities which permanently alter gross brain morphology
(Dobbing 1974). Except for the granular cells of the cerebellum, and perhaps some in the forebrain, the adult number
of neurones is reached in mid-gestation before the precursors
of other types of brain cells begin to divide rapidly (Dobbing & Smart 1974). A minor reduction in the number of neurones is probably not important functionally. A second spurt
in the number of brain cells begins at about 30 weeks of gestation and continues until the age of 2 years (Dobbing &
Sands 1973). This increase in macroglia provides many more
brain cells than the earlier spurt in the number of neurones
(Dobbing & Sands 1970). Most of these glial cells are oligodendroglia which can develop in adulthood also (Warwick &
Williams 1973), indicating that a reduction in their usual
rate of formation may not be functionally serious.

Usually the degree of myelination in the central nervous system is estimated from the total lipid content (Dobbing & Sands 1973). The total lipid content changes little during the first few months of gestation; thereafter, the lipid concentration of the gray matter increases rapidly to reach adult levels at about 3 months of age. The lipid concentration of the white matter also increases rapidly during the first year after birth but it decreases by 2 years of age when it is about 90% of the adult value. There is no information about the myelination of specific tracts in the living that could be useful for the analysis of possible catch-up growth.

During postnatal development the bodies of neurones enlarge, particularly the cytoplasm. There are increases in Nissl substance, branching of axons and apical dendrites, and the formation of basal dendrites (Dodge et al. 1975). Buell and Coleman (1979) have reported elongation and increased branching of terminal apical dendrites of parahippocampal cells between 51 and 80 years of age. These findings indicate a potential for growth persists throughout life.

Retardation in Malnourished Children

The age at which malnutrition occurs is very important in relation to its effects on the brain (Rosso, Hormazábal & Winick 1970). Consequently, studies of experimental animals must be interpreted in relation to differences among species in the timing of the rapid phase of growth in brain weight relative to birth (Dobbing 1974). The pig and man are similar in this respect. The effects of prenatal malnutrition are of particular interest. The brain appears relatively protected against malnutrition until about the 30th week of gestation but growth retardation during the last trimester results in a small brain with a reduced number of cells (Winick & Rosso 1969). In children with intrauterine growth retardation the brain is small for gestational age and contains fewer cells than normal (Sarma & Rao 1974). Information is lacking in regard to the effects on specific cell types and on the development of cell processes and synapses.

Head circumference is small in children malnourished before the age of 2 years (Graham & Adrianzen 1971). Some of this deficit is due to a thin scalp and cranial vault (Engsner, Shoadagne, Sjögren & Vahlquist 1974). There is increased subarachnoid fluid which is responsible for an

increased transillumination of the head (Mönckeberg 1975) but
the ventricles are normal in size (Engsner et al. 1974). In
such malnourished children the brain is small with high correlations between head circumference and brain weight
(Winick & Rosso 1969).

Some data show malnourished children catch up in head
circumference if they are treated before the age of 4 months
but contrary data have been reported. The differences between reports reflect the nature of the rehabilitation.
Others have shown catch-up in head circumference even when
malnutrition occurs as late as 5 years of age if there is
excellent rehabilitation (Branko 1979).

The younger the malnourished child at death, the greater
the effect of malnutrition on brain size and brain cell number (Winick & Rosso 1969). The brains of infants dying of
malnutrition during the first year of life are reduced about
15% in weight and cell number but cell size is considered
normal (Winick & Rosso 1969). The reduction in cell number
is about 40% in low birth weight infants who die of malnutrition during the first year. These infants have only about
40% of the normal number of brain cells. Probably the reduction is in macroglia rather than neurones except in the
cerebellum where both types of cells are less numerous than
normal (Winick 1970). Myelination is retarded but there are
no apparent abnormalities in the composition of myelin or
the amount of myelin per cell (Fishman, Prensky & Dodge 1969).

Malnutrition after the age of 2 years has little effect
on the number of neurones but it causes a deficit in the
number of macroglia. The importance of this in relation to
cognitive development is unclear. For rehabilitation from
malnutrition to be effective in regard to the development
and growth of the brain, it must occur early enough during
cellular proliferation to allow catch-up (Winick 1970). If
the malnutrition occurs after the age of 2 years the deficits
in cell number and myelination persist despite rehabilitation
but the increased transillumination and deficits in cell
size are reversible (Dodge et al. 1975).

Catch-up in Pathological States

Studies of catch-up growth in malnourished children during rehabilitation are made difficult by the effects of many

intervening variables (including inadequate rehabilitation) and the lack of appropriate controls. Consequently, some have studied children in good socioeconomic circumstances but with intrauterine growth retardation or diseases that interfere with postnatal nutrition. The latter studies have included children with malabsorption as a result of conditions such as cystic fibrosis. Extraordinarily rapid and marked catch-up growth in head size occurs in some of these children (Bray & Herbst 1973). The catch-up in head circumference may be associated with marked separation of the sutures due to an increase in intracranial pressure. There is papilledema in some cases (Marks, Borns, Steg, Stine, Stroud & Vates 1978) but not in others (De Levie & Nogrady 1970). In the latter group it must be assumed the increased intracranial pressure, while sufficient to cause sutural separation, was too slight to cause other signs of increased intracranial pressure.

The rapid head enlargement and increased intracranial pressure observed in these children is probably due to a rapid increase in brain size. Marks and others (1978) reported data for two brothers, aged 2.5 and 4 years, with deprivation dwarfism. Their head circumferences increased very rapidly, in association with sutural separation, after hospitalization. Computerized axial tomography (CAT) scans show enlargement of the brain obliterated the shadows of the ventricular system and of the longitudinal cerebral fissure in each boy.

In summary, the study of children fully rehabilitated from malnutrition has shown surprisingly rapid increases in brain size at ages up to 5 years. It is possible that catch-up growth could occur at even older ages were it not for interlocking of cranial sutures which prevents rapid brain enlargement.

REFERENCES

Apfelbaum M, Brigant L, Duret F (1973). Relationship between the age of appearance of obesity and adipocyte diameter in 256 obese and 57 non-obese women. In "The Regulation of the Adipose Tissue Mass." Marseilles: Proc IV Int Meet Endocrinol, p 215.
Ashworth A (1969). Growth rates in children recovering from protein calorie malnutrition. Br J Nutr 23:835.

Björntorp P, Sjöström L (1971). The number and size of adipose tissue fat cells in relation to metabolism in human obesity. Metabolism 20:703.

Branko Z (1979). Height, weight, and head circumference in survivors of marasmus and kwashiorkor. Am J Clin Nutr 32: 1719.

Bray PF, Herbst JJ (1973). Pseudotumor cerebri as a sign of "catch-up" growth in cystic fibrosis. Am J Dis Child 126:78.

Brook CGD (1972). Evidence for a sensitive period in adipose cell replication in man. Lancet ii:624.

Buell SJ, Coleman PD (1979). Dendritic growth in the aged human brain and failure of growth in senile dementia. Science 206:854.

De Levie M, Nogrady MB (1970). Rapid brain growth upon restoration of adequate nutrition causing false radiographic evidence of increased intracranial pressure. J Pediatr 76: 523.

Dobbing J (1968). Effects of experimental undernutrition on development of the nervous system. In Scrimshaw NS, Gordon JE (eds): "Malnutrition, Learning and Behaviour," Cambridge, Mass: M.I.T. Press, p 181.

Dobbing J (1974). The later growth of the brain and its vulnerability. Pediatrics 53:2.

Dobbing J, Sands J (1970). Timing of neuroblast multiplication in developing human brain. Nature 226:639.

Dobbing J, Sands J (1973). Quantitative growth and development of human brain. Arch Dis Child 48:757.

Dobbing J, Smart JL (1974). Vulnerability of developing brain and behaviour. Br Med Bull 30:164.

Dodge PR, Prensky AL, Feigin RD (1975). "Nutrition and the Developing Nervous System." St. Louis: Mosby, p 312.

Engsner G, Shoadagne B, Sjögren I, Vahlquist B (1974). Brain growth in children with marasmus. A study using head circumference measurement, transillumination and ultrasonic echo ventriculography. Ups J Med Sci 79:116.

Fishman MA, Prensky AL, Dodge PL (1969). Low content of cerebral lipids in infants suffering from malnutrition. Nature 221:552.

Graham GG, Adrianzen BT (1971). Growth, inheritance and environment. Pediatr Res 5:691.

Gurr MI, Kirtland J (1978). Adipose tissue cellularity: a review. 1. Techniques for studying cellularity. Int J Obesity 2:401.

Häger A (1977). Adipose cell size and number in relation to obesity. Postgrad Med J 53:101.

Häger A, Sjöström L, Arvidsson B, Björntorp P, Smith U (1977).
Body fat and adipose tissue cellularity in infants--a
longitudinal study. Metabolism 26:607.

Hernesniemi I, Zachmann M, Prader A (1974). Skinfold thickness in infancy and adolescence. A longitudinal correlation study in normal children. Helv Paediatr Acta 29:523.

Hirsch J, Knittle JL (1970). Cellularity of obese and non-
obese human adipose tissue. Fed Proc 29:1516.

Lemonnier D (1972). Effect of age, sex and site on the cellularity of the adipose tissue in mice and rats rendered
obese by a high fat diet. J Clin Invest 51:2907.

Marks HG, Borns P, Steg NL, Stine SB, Stroud HH, Vates TS
(1978). Catch-up brain growth--demonstration by CAT scan.
J Pediatr 93:254.

Mönckeberg F (1975). The effect of malnutrition on physical
growth and brain development. In Prescott JW, Read MS,
Coursin DB (eds): "Brain Function and Malnutrition:
Neuropsychological Methods of Assessment," New York: John
Wiley & Sons, p 15.

Rosso P, Hormazábal J, Winick M (1970). Changes in brain
weight, cholesterol, phospholipid, and DNA content in
marasmic children. Am J Clin Nutr 23:1275.

Salans LB, Horton ES, Sims EAH (1971). Experimental obesity
in man; cellular character of adipose tissue. J Clin
Invest 50:1005.

Sarma MKJ, Rao KS (1974). Biochemical composition of different regions in brains of small-for-date infants. J Neurochem 22:671.

Wachholder A (1976). Poids et taille des enfants, en fonction
de l'alimentation précoce, dans l'énchantillon de Bruxelles.
In "Compte-Rendu de la XIII Réunion des Equipes Chargées
des Etudes sur la Croissance et le Développement de
l'enfant Normal." Rennes: Centre International de
L'enfance, p 48.

Warwick R, Williams PL (eds; 1973). "Gray's Anatomy." (35th
British ed). Philadelphia: Saunders, p 779.

Widdowson EM, Shaw WT (1973). Full and empty fat cells.
Lancet ii:905.

Winick M (1970). Cellular growth in intrauterine malnutrition. Pediatr Clin North Am 17:69.

Winick M, Noble A (1966). Cellular response in rats during
malnutrition at various ages. J Nutr 89:300.

Winick M, Rosso P (1969). Head circumference and cellular
growth of the brain in normal and marasmic children. J
Pediatr 74:774.

Winick M, Brasel JA, Rosso P (1972). Nutrition and cell
growth. Curr Concepts Nutr 1:49.

Index

PROGRESS IN CLINICAL AND BIOLOGICAL RESEARCH